Antimicrobial Activity of Lactoferrin and Lactoferrin Derived Peptides

ANTIMICROBIAL ACTIVITY OF LACTOFERRIN AND LACTOFERRIN DERIVED PEPTIDES

HÅVARD JENSSEN

Nova Science Publishers, Inc.
New York

For permission to use material from this book please contact us:
Telephone 631-231-7269; Fax 631-231-8175
Web Site: http://www.novapublishers.com

LIBRARY OF CONGRESS CATALOGING-IN-PUBLICATION DATA

ISBN: 978-1-60692-518-8

Available upon request

Published by Nova Science Publishers, Inc. ✢ New York

CONTENTS

PREFACE

Milk is a vital nutritional source for offspring of all mammals, including humans. In addition to its nutritional value it is a rich source of proteins, of which lactoferrin (Lf) is one. Lf is truly a multifunctional molecule which has been studied extensively over the past decades. It is best known for its ability to bind iron, which initially leads to the discovery of its antibacterial activity. In addition, Lf has demonstrated potent antiviral, antifungal and antiparasitic activity, towards a spectrum of strains. Additionally, it has been evaluated as an important host defense molecule during infant development. Extensive work has been done to characterize the active domains in Lf, testing numerous Lf-derived peptides and related peptide libraries for activity towards different microbes. The peptides structural requirements for antimicrobial activity has been addressed, and compared to other cationic host defense peptides which related chemical and biological characteristics, in an attempt to understand different antimicrobial modes of action.

The antimicrobial activity of Lf and one N-terminal peptide fragment of Lf (lactoferricin) are the main topics of this chapter, with particular focus on antiviral activities. Antibacterial, –fungal and –parasitic acitivity will also be discussed, in addition to the selective activity demonstrated by Lf and lactoferricin, towards tumor cell membranes. It has also become increasingly recognized that several antimicrobial protein and peptides possesses immunomodulatory activity, thus these properties will be discussed in brief detail.

Chapter 1

INTRODUCTION

Antimicrobial peptides are produced by a wide variety of organisms as their first line of defense [127], and are found in large quantities in all secretory fluids. They are typically relatively short (12 to 100 amino acids), positively charged (net +2 to +9), amphiphilic, and have been isolated from single-celled microorganisms, amphibians, birds, fish, plants and mammals, including man [117, 388]. To date, hundreds of such peptides have been isolated [128], indicating their importance in the innate immune system [129]. The most prominent peptide structures are 2-4 β-strands, amphipathic α-helices, loop structures and extended structures [40, 44]. These peptides tend to have a direct effect on the microbe, such as damaging or destabilizing the bacterial, viral, or fungal membrane, but their involvement in the orchestration of the innate immune– and inflammatory response has also been demonstrated [66, 127, 129]. They are also able to enhance phagocytosis, stimulate prostaglandin release, neutralize the septic effects of bacterial lipopolysaccharide, promote recruitment and accumulation of various immune cells at inflammatory sites [95, 405], promote angiogenesis [186] and induce wound-repair [59]. Antimicrobial peptides of mammalian origin have also been demonstrated to have an active role in the transition to the adaptive immune response by being chemotactic for human monocytes [348] and T cells [66] and by exhibiting adjuvant and polarizing effects in influencing dendritic cell development [76].

The most abundant antimicrobial proteins include lactoferrin, lysozyme, and collectin [52, 209]. The antimicrobial activity of these types of proteins is related to bacterial lysis or opsonization of the pathogen. For example, mannose-binding proteins interacting with HIV [138] and neutralization of influenza A virus by surfactant protein A [33]. Lactoferrin is known to work as an opsonin for bacterial clearance [176], but this activity has not been illustrated for viruses.

The following chapter will provide an overview of the (direct) antimicrobial functions of the milk protein lactoferrin (Lf) and one of its most studied pepsin derived peptides, lactoferricin (Lfcin). The effect of other derivatives of lactoferrin will also be discussed in less detail. The antimicrobial activity will comprise; antiviral, antibacterial, antifungal and antiparasitic activity. Both Lf and Lfcin has been shown to target lipid membranes, thus antitumor activity will also be discussed. The chapter will conclude with a discussion of some novel applications of Lf and Lfcin.

LACTOFERRIN – AN IMPORTANT WHEY PROTEIN

Dairy products and in particular milk is a rich and important sorce of protein, fat, minerals (e.g. Ca^{2+}, P^{3+}, Na^{+}, K^{+}, Mg^{2+} and Zn^{2+}) and vitamins (e.g. Riboflavin, B_{12} and A) in the human diaet [157]. Some milk proteins and their cleavage products have turned out to represent more than just mere nutrients. In bovine milk, for example, the protein fraction constitutes about 3.5%, and of this fraction about 80% is casein and the remaining 20% is whey protein [401]. Whey is sepereated out as a by-product during the cheese making process and contains all the essential amino acids. One important whey protein is lactoferrin (Lf), and it constitutes about 2-3% of the whey fraction which equals 0.2mg/mL in bovine milk [206]. Secretion of Lf in to the milk has also been documented in a variety of other mammals (horse, buffalo, camel, goat, pig, guinea-pig, mare, mouse, rhesus monkey and human) [77, 182, 196, 228, 229, 309], at concentrations at least ten times higher than in bovine milk.

Lactoferrin (Lf) is an 80 kDa multifunctional, neutrophil-derived, monomeric glycoprotein [51], distributed in the secondary granules of polynuclear lymphocytes and secreted from various exocrine glands [19, 230], thus explaining the high concentrations of Lf in milk and on mucosal surface [227]. The protein folds into two homologous globular lobes linked with an 11 amino acid α-helix [21]. In human lactoferrin (hLf) this equals N-lobe $^{1\text{-}332}$, α-helix hinge-region $^{333\text{-}343}$ and C-lobe $^{344\text{-}703}$ (figure 1) [8]. Each lobe may reversibly bind one ferric ion (Fe^{3+}) [22]. In fact, Lf binds iron with much higher affinity and stability than the plasma iron-transport protein transferrin [22, 389], though these proteins share many structural and functional features [21]. Lf evolved several million years ago and its importance as an antimicrobial protein is underscored by numerous conserved gene segments.

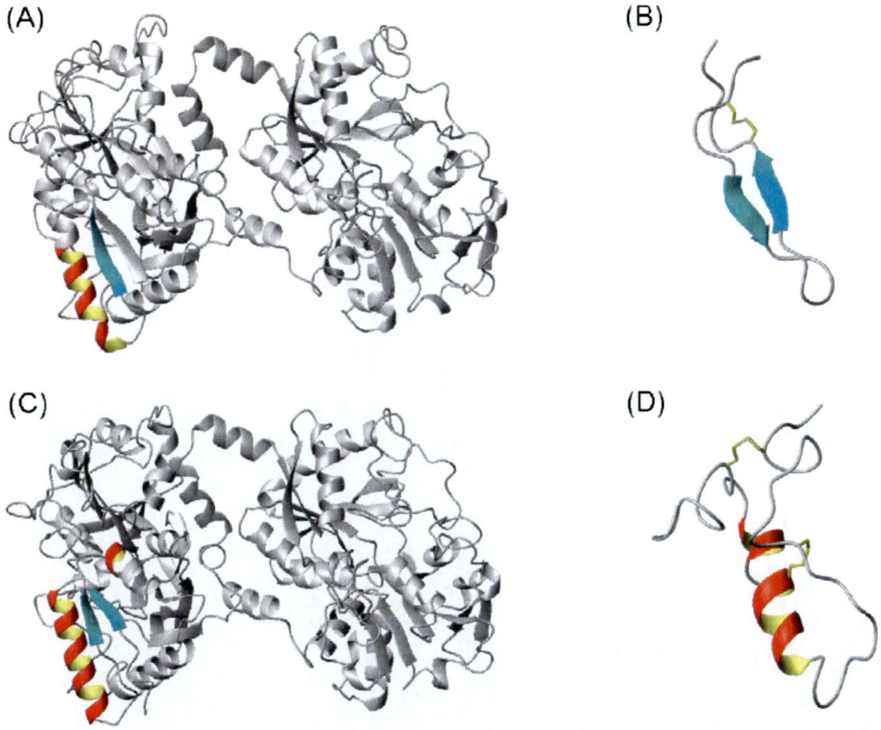

Figure 1. Lactoferrin and lactoferricin structures. (A) Bovine lactoferrin (PDB code 1BLF) [244], the colored segment corresponding to the LfcinB sequence, (B) bovine lactoferricin (PDB code 1LFC) [158] after pepsin digestion from bLf [219], (C) human lactoferrin (PDB code 1LFG) [254], the colored segment corresponding to the LfcinH sequence [281] and (D) human lactoferricin (PDB code 1Z6V) [155] after pepsin digestion from hLf [238]. The disulfide bonds in LfcinB and LfcinH are indicated in yellow and the figures have been prepared with use of the graphic program MolMol 2K.1 [189].

The conserved regions namely comprise areas on the surface of the protein structure [105]. There is 69% sequence homology between the bovine and the human Lf (bLf and hLf) [274, 289]. Lf can be isolated from several mammals, and the high homology is further underlined by aligning the N-terminal fragments of Lf from the different species (table 1). Lf is also resistant to tryptic digestion, resulting in partial survival following passage through the gastrointestinal tract [48]. One of the main physiological functions of Lf is to bind iron, which initially

Table 1. N-terminal fragments of Lf from different species

Origin	Amino acid sequence (single letter code)																							
Human	GRRRRS	V	Q	WC$_1$	AV	S	QP	E	AT	KC$_2$	FQ	W	Q	RN	MRR	VRG	P	P	V	S	C$_2$	IKR	DSPIQ	C$_1$
Bovine	APRKN	V	R	WC$_1$	TI	S	QP	E	WF	KC$_2$	RR	W	Q	WR	MKK	LGA	P	S	I	T	C$_2$	VRR	AFALE	C$_1$
Porcine	APKKG	V	R	WC$_1$	VI	S	TA	E	YS	KC$_2$	RQ	W	Q	SK	IRR	TN-	P	-	I	F	C$_2$	IRR	ASPTD	C$_1$
Buffalo	APRKN	V	R	WC$_1$	TI	S	QP	E	WL	KC$_2$	HR	W	Q	WR	MKK	LGA	P	S	I	T	C$_2$	VRR	AFVLE	C$_1$
Caprine	APRKN	V	R	WC$_1$	AI	S	PP	E	GS	KC$_2$	YQ	W	Q	RR	MRK	LGA	P	S	I	T	C$_2$	VRR	TSALE	C$_1$
Camel	ASKKS	V	R	WC$_1$	TT	S	PA	E	SS	KC$_2$	AQ	W	Q	RR	MKK	VRG	P	S	V	T	C$_2$	VKK	TSRFE	C$_1$
Equine	APRKS	V	R	WC$_1$	TI	S	PA	E	AA	KC$_2$	AK	F	Q	RN	MKK	VRG	P	S	V	S	C$_2$	IRK	TSSFE	C$_1$
Rat	RIDTV	V	R	WC$_1$	TI	S	RN	E	AQ	KC$_2$	FM	W	Q	EM	LNK	AGV	P	K	L	R	C$_2$	ARK	YFMPH	C$_1$
Mouse	AKATT	V	R	WC$_1$	AV	S	NS	E	EE	KC$_2$	LR	W	Q	NE	MRK	VGG	p	P	L	S	C$_2$	VKK	SSTRQ	C$_1$

The amino acid sequence of the N-terminal part of several Lf molecules are compared and segregated into homologues regions. Information regarding the different sequences has been collected from NCBI GenBank, given in brackets and the Lf types are from; human (AAW71443), bovine (P24627), porcine (NP_999527), buffalo (O77698), caprine (AAV92908), camel (Q9TUM0), equine (O77811), rat (XP_236657), and mouse (P08071) origin. The solid boxes indicate identical residues, while the doted lines indicate residues with similar biochemical properties. The horizontal lines in porcine Lf indicate amino acid deletions. Positively charge amino acid residues are color-coded in blue, while negatively charge residues are colored red. Cysteines forming disulfide bonds are numbered with subscript numbers to indicate their pairing.

was identified as a feature of the protein contributing to its antibacterial activity, by sequestering iron, a necessary nutritional requirement for most bacterial pathogens. Thus inhibiting bacterial growth of a broad spectrum of bacterial strains [16, 54, 101, 104]. Lf can also inhibit viral infections [25, 35, 85, 132, 135, 160, 210, 221, 222, 284, 334, 345, 371]. Antiviral activity of Lf functions against both naked [14, 223, 300, 334], and enveloped viruses [7, 85, 111, 134, 135, 161, 221, 222, 246, 279, 284, 337, 412], and the activity is exerted during an early phase of the viral infection. Lf from several species possesses antiviral activity towards different human viruses, although bLf is often reported to exhibit higher antiviral activity than hLf [5, 7, 210, 221]. Iron saturation does not appear to influence the antiviral activity [222, 284, 345] in contrast to its antibacterial activity. In addition, Lf inhibits tumor growth [360], fungal infections [184, 323] and parasitic infection [392]. Several immunological functions are also ascribed to Lf, although their detailed mechanisms remain unknown [50, 71, 116, 304, 307, 380].

Due to advances in processing technologies, industrial production of different products with varying protein contents from liquid whey is available. Today, single proteins like lactoferrin, are isolated and purified from whey in a cost efficient manner by several companies e.g. DMV international (Netherlands), Morinaga milk industries (Japan), or produced recombinantly by companies like DSM Pharmaceutical Products (Netherlands), Agennix (USA) and Pharming AM (Netherlands).

FRAGMENTS OF LACTOFERRIN

Several separate studies have been conducted to identify the domains of Lf contributing to its antimicrobial activity. In most of these studies Lf has been digested with commercial enzymes such as pepsin, trypsin and chymotrypsin isolated from pig pancreas [351]. However, the significance of the peptide fragments, generated with these enzymes, on the human gut flora, and whether or not Lf is degradable in the gastrointestinal tract with human enzymes have been debated. Thus, it could be argued that the search for antimicrobial peptide fragment from Lf digestion should have been done with use of human gastric- and duodenal enzymes [29]. To investigate the resistance of Lf to enzymatic digestion in the gut Brittan *et al.* [49] examined the gastric fluid from 12 milk fed infants, concluding that Lf was fare more resistant to digestion, compared to other milk proteins like transferrin and casein [49]. Interestingly the enzymatic degradation of Lf was also very sensitive to changes in the pH, thus postprandial (the digestive period after a meal) pH in the gut decrease Lf degradation [49]. It has also been demonstrated that Lf from different species has variable sensitivity for enzymatic degradation [3, 48]. bLf degradation has also been investigated in an murine *in vivo* model, demonstrating that bLf partially survived through the gastrointestinal tract, and fractions of the protein was degraded into larger fragments, that still contained intact receptor binding regions and the antimicrobial active centre [198].

Studies investigating different hydrolysates of Lf have lead to the discovery of multiple peptide fragments with antimicrobial activity against specific pathogens (table 2). The most investigated peptide has been isolated from the N-terminal domain of Lf, following pepsin treatment [351], and the peptide is termed lactoferricin (Lfcin). Bovine lactoferricin (LfcinB) is comprised of bLf $^{17-41}$, while human lactoferricin (LfcinH) consists of two fragments, amino acid residue 1 to 11 and residue 12 to 47, connected by a disulfide bridge [30]. Reproduction of these results however has been difficult, and several recent publications defines LfcinB as bLf $^{17-42}$ [83], and LfcinH as a single fragment of hLf $^{1-49}$ (figure 2) [155]. LfcinB features a loop region attributable to a disulfide bridge between residues 19 and 36, a region which is also found in the homologous region of LfcinH (amino acid residues 20 and 37) [30]. Both LfcinB and LfcinH create a surface-exposed amphipathic α-helical domain in Lf, prior to pepsin digestion (figure 1) [20, 133, 259]. In addition, the larger LfcinH comprises a parallel β-sheet structure. After pepsin cleavage, LfcinB loses its α-helical domain and becomes a distorted twisted antiparallel β-sheet [158], whereas LfcinH retains its α-helical domain but loses its β-sheet [155].

Lfcin has been shown to excrete antibacterial activity against a wide selection of bacterial, viral, and fungal pathogens, as well as some protozoa [167, 354, 378, 387]. The peptide has also demonstrated quite high selectivity for tumor cell membranes over healthy cells, thereby possessing antitumor activity [119]. The biological properties of Lfcin will be discussed later in greater detail, in individual sections.

Pepsin digestion of Lf has also generated other peptide fragments e.g. the lactoferrampin, lactoferroxin, an anti-aggregating peptide and a cell-adhesion motif peptide. In brief lactoferrampin was identified after a sequence scan of bLf, based on knowledge of common features for antimicrobial peptides. The peptide fragment of lactoferrampin (Lfampin) corresponds to bLf $^{268-284}$ (table 2) [368]. The peptide has demonstrated a substantially higher anti-candida activity than bLf, in addition to a broad-spectrum antibacterial activity, not completely identical to that of LfcinB [368]. Quantitative structure activity relation studies of Lfampin and its anti-candida activity have also been conducted. The results concluded that Lfampin exerted its candidacidal activity through a cluster of positively charged residues at the peptides C-terminal end in combination with a α-helical facilitating N-terminal domain [369].

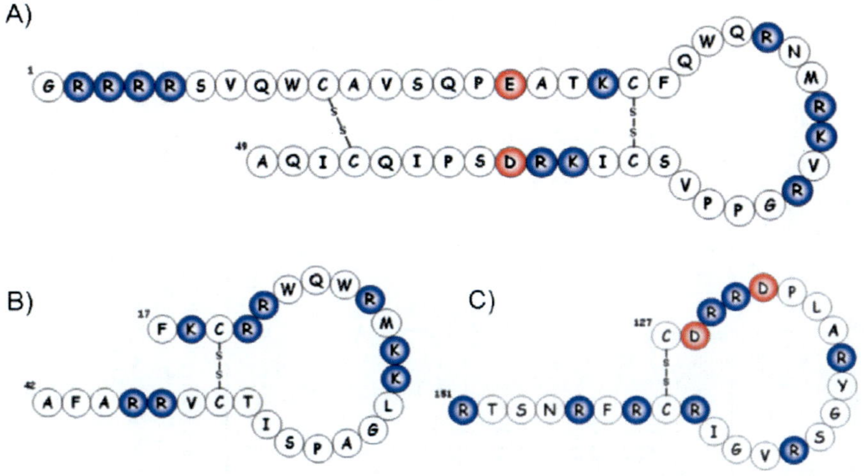

Figure 2. Peptide projections. Primary structure projection of LfcinH consisting of amino acid residues 1 to 49 (A), LfcinB comprising residues 17 to 42 (B) and the heparan sulfate binding loop of gC HSV-1 from residue 127 to 151 (C). The cationic residues are coloured blue while anionic residues are labelled in red. The figure is reprinted and modified from reference [167], with permission from Cellular and Molecular Life Sciences, Copyright © 2005, Birkhäuser Verlag AG.

Another group of peptide fragments from Lf have been termed lactoferroxins. Three different elements of hLf have been isolated, (Tyr-Leu-Gly-Ser-Gly-Tyr-OCH_3, Arg-Tyr-Tyr-Gly-Tyr-OCH_3 and Lys-Tyr-Leu-Gly-Pro-Gln-Tyr-OCH_3), corresponding to the metyl esters of hLf $^{318-323}$, hLf $^{536-540}$ and hLf $^{673-679}$, respectively (table 2) [347]. The lactoferroxins have been classified as opioide peptides, which mimic the effect of opiates, referred to as alkaloids found in opium. Opioide peptides have earlier also been isolated from enzymatic hydrolysates of major milk proteins like α–casein [213, 423] and casomorphins (a precursor to α– and β –casein) [47, 144].

Table 2. Selected examples of biological active fragments Lf from different species

Peptide	Primary amino acid sequence	Charge [a]	pI [b]	Hydrophilicity[c]	Hydrophilicity ratio [%] [d]	GRAVY[e]	References
LfcinB $^{17-42}$	$FKC_1RRWQWRMKKLGAPSITC_1VRRAFA$	7.9	12.2	0.1	38	-0.485	[30, 155, 167]
LfcinB $^{17-30}$	FKC RRWQWRMKKLG	6	12.1	0.3	50	-1.421	
Deca-peptide	FKC RRWQWRM	4	12.1	0.1	50	-1.550	[362]
Hexa-peptide	$RRWRWR\text{-}CONH_2$	5	14.0	0.9	67	-3.300	[352]
hLfH $^{1-11}$	$GRRRRSVQWC_1A$	4	12.4	0.6	55	-1.373	[249]
LfcinH $^{1-49}$	$GRRRRSVQWC_1AVSQPEATKC_2FQWQR$ $NMRRVRGPPVSC_2IKRDSPIQC_1IQA$	8.8	11.9	0.3	49	-0.863	[30, 155, 167]
hLf $^{18-42}$	$TKC_1FQWQRNMRRVRGPPVSC_1IKRDS$	5.9	11.8	0.4	52	-1.140	[155]
LfcinC $^{14-42}$	$PEWSKC_1YQWQRRMRKLGAPSITC_1VRRTSA$	5.9	11.3	0.2	45	-0.976	[287]
LfcinM $^{17-41}$	$EKC_1LRWQEMLNKAGGPPLSC_1VKKSS$	2.9	9.7	0.3	48	-0.684	[382]
LfcinP $^{17-41}$	$SKC_1RQWQSKIRRTNPIFC_1IRRASPT$	6.9	12.2	0.3	52	-1.024	[382]
pLf $^{18-37}$	$KC_1RQWQSKIRRTNPIFC_1IRR$	6.9	12.2	0.4	55	-1.175	[64]
Lactoferroxin hLF $^{318-323}$	YLGSGY	0	5.9	-1.0	17	-0.067	[347]
Lactoferroxin hLf $^{536-540}$	RYYGY	1	9.4	-0,8	20	-1.760	[347]
Lactoferroxin hLf $^{673-679}$	KYLGPQY	1	9.5	-0,5	29	-1.171	[347]
Lfampin bLf $_{268-284}$	WKLLSKAQEKFGKNKSR	5	11.1	0.7	65	-1.482	[368]

dNote: Amino acid sequence is given in single letter code. Cysteines forming disulfide bonds are numbered with subscript numbers to indicate their pairing, the cationic residues are highlighted. (a) Net positive charge at pH 7.0, (b) Iso-electric point, (c) The average hydrophilicity in the peptide, (d) The ratio of hydrophilic residues over the total number of residues and (e) Grand average of hydrophaticity [199]. All chemical properties of the peptides have been calculated with use of the Peptide Property Calculater, a free-ware provide by Innovagen AB (Lund, Sween), except GRAVY which is calculated using services at ExPASy ProtPharm tool, provided by the Swiss Institute of Bioinformatics.

Sakamoto *et al.* [295] used a random hexameric peptide library of the Lf sequence to identify two peptides containing a short motif of Arg-Gly-Asp (RGD-motif). Similar motifs have also been described in synthetic peptides derived from fibronectin, an important extracellular matrix glycoprotein involved in platelet aggregation. The fibrionectin derived peptides containing these RGD-motifs have demonstrated to interfere with platelet aggregation [78, 108]. Further experiments have also demonstrated that Lf interacts with fibronectin, indicating that one function of hLf is to block various interactions between cell surface and adhesion molecules [295]. Another short tetra-peptide has also been derived from hLf corresponding to the sequence $hLf^{39\text{-}42}$ (Lys-Arg-Asp-Ser). This peptide has also demonstrated the ability to inhibit adenosine diphosphate (ADP)-induced platelet aggregation [233], despite little resemblance with RGD motif.

Chapter 2

Antiviral Activity of LF

The antiviral activity of Lf has been investigated in great detail. Initially it was thought that only enveloped viruses were affected, and that this activity was due to either inhibition of virus host interaction e.g; hepatitis B virus (HBV), herpes simplex virus (HSV) and human cytomegalovirus (HCMV) [6, 132, 135] or direct interaction between Lf and the viral particle e.g; feline herpes virus (FHV-1), hepatitis C virus (HCV), hepatitis G virus (HGV) and human immunodeficiency virus (HIV) [25, 34, 160, 161]. Lately naked viruses e.g.; rota-, polio-, adeno- and entero-virus [14, 210, 223, 276, 333], have also been demonstrated to be susceptible for inhibition by Lf. In all cases studied, it appears that Lf exhibits its antiviral activity at an early phase in the infection process [6, 14, 25, 34, 35, 132, 161, 210, 223, 276, 333, 383]. *In vitro* studies have also demonstrated that Lf exhibits synergy in combination with zidovudine against HIV-1 [373]. A synergistic antiviral activity has also been observed for HSV-1 and HSV-2 when acyclovir was used in combination with Lf [5, 168]. Additionally, Lf have been shown to possess antiviral activity towards acyclovir resistant clinical isolates [5].

Antiviral Mode of Action of LF

To investigate the antiviral mode of action of Lf, a broad panel of experimental assays has been developed. Pre-incubation of Lf with the host cell appears to be essential for the proteins antiviral activity towards a specter of viruses, e.g. HBV, HS-adapted Sindbis – and Semliki Forest virus, HCMV, HSV-1 and HSV-2 [6, 132, 135, 383]. Expression of early and late HCMV antigens, as well as production of infectious viral progeny, was effectively inhibited by Lf from different species [7]. The activity was associated with the proteins moiety but not its iron molecule or sialic acid. Time of addition studies demonstrated that 5 to 10 minutes pre-incubation of Lf with the host cell was sufficient to prevent HCMV infection, even when removing Lf after addition of the virus [135]. Complementing studies demonstrated that Lf possessed no activity against HCMV, if added after viral penetration, thus concluding that the activity was at the level of virus adsorption or penetration [134].

In addition to this, Andersen *et al.* [6] showed that the antiviral activity of Lf not was improved by pre-incubation of Lf with HSV-1 or HSV-2 prior to infection, indicating that the antiviral activity of Lf must be exerted through interaction with a cellular target, rather than a target on the viral particle itself [6]. Conversely, Marchetti *et al.* [221, 222] suggested that Lf prevents HSV entry in part by binding to the virus particles. However these mechanisms need not be exclusive, and may reflect the different experimental conditions. Electron micrographs have confirmed that Lf must be located at the cell surface to exert antiviral activity against HSV [6].These and others studies have also demonstrated that Lf remains at the cell surface after exposure [293], which explains the post-infection effect of Lf observed with the plaque reduction assay with HSV on Vero cells [6].

Lf inhibition of viral infections by interfering with virus-host cell interaction, are likely to involve commen host cell surface molecules. Proteoglycans are found in all types of tissue, in intracellular granule secretions [187], extracellular matrix [162], and on the cell surface [37]. Proteoglycans consist of a core protein and one or more covalently attached glycosaminoglycan chains. The degree of sulfation in the glycosaminoglycan molecules makes them among the most anionic compounds present on mammalian cell surfaces [357]. This strong net negative charge permits glycosaminoglycan to bind to small cations [268], proteins [159], enzymes [273] growth factors [82, 185, 216], cytokines [56], chemokines [150] and lipoproteins [211, 262], in addition to a number of pathogens, including viruses [240, 326].

Host cell infection by several viral pathogens has been shown to be highly dependent on these glycosaminoglycan molecules on the host cell surface. One of the most prominent glycosaminoglycan molecules for virus interaction is heparan sulfate [240, 326]. Lf is known to have high net charge and two N-terminal domains for glycosaminoglycan binding [220, 310, 396], thus it has been demonstrated that Lf can bind to heparan sulfate with rather high affinity [169]. Additionally, viral entry of HSV-1 is effectively blocked by Lf [6], most likely as a result of Lf interaction with cell surface heparan sulfate [135, 221, 224]. Anti-

HSV activity of Lf has been investigated with several cell lines, both deficient in- and expressing different glycosaminoglycan molecules at the cell surface. The results have shown that heparan sulfate at the cell surface is important for Lf to exert antiviral activity against HSV [6, 224]. HSV-1 and HSV-2 differ in their interaction with heparan sulfate [146], which may explain the different antiviral activity of Lf towards the two viruses [5]. Similar results have been shown for heparan sulfate -adapted Sindbis and Semliki Forest virus, where their ability to infect BHK-21 cells effectively could be blocked by Lf, while non-adopted viruses not were affected [383].

When Lf was either pre-incubated with the cells prior to infection (4 hours at 37°C), or added after viral attachment (1 hour at 4°C), there was no detectable difference in its ability to block viral entry [6]. It has also been demonstrated that Lf needs to be at the cell surface to block viral entry, and after 4 hours incubation of Lf with the cells, a significant amount of Lf was internalized. Thus indicating that the cells were able to adapt a long lasting antiviral immunity after exposure to Lf. Similar immunity to HSV infection, lasting for several hours, have also been reported for derivatives of dispirotripiperazine [299], interacting with heparan sulfate.

However, not all viruses required heparan sulfate as an attachment receptor on the host cell. Hantavirus infection of Vero E6 cells results in formation of foci, and the number of focies evaluated 5 days post infection was significantly reduced when the cells were treated with Lf. Pretreatment of the cells with Lf increased its activity. However, by washing the monolayer with PBS after Lf pretreatment, the antiviral activity was reduced [246]. Suggested that Lf was able to block hantavirus infection through a weak interaction between a host cell molecule and Lf, implying that heparan sulfate not was the target molecule for Lf in this hantavirus model.

Another crucial target for Lf is obviously the viral particle itself. HCV infection of PH5CH8 cells were effectively inhibited by pre-incubation of bLf with the viral particle, prior to infection. Conversely, pretreatment of the PH5CH8 cells with bLf had no effect on the viral infection rate, suggesting that bLf exerted its anti-HCV activity through direct interaction with the viral particle [161]. Both hLf and bLf have also been demonstrated to directly interact with two envelope proteins in HCV, E1 and E2 [412]. Similar direct interaction between Lf and the virus particle has been demonstrated for HIV, where Lf strongly interacts with the V3 loop of envelope protein gp120. Thus it has been hypothesized that shielding of this domain results in inhibition of HIV fusion and entry into MT4 cells [337]. Both HIV-1 replication and syncytium (giant cell) formation could also be inhibited in a dose dependent manner by Lf, and the effect was not dependent on

Lf being either in its apo- or holo-form [284]. Supporting studies have demonstrated that bLf can block viral infection of HIV-1 using either CXCR4- or CCR5-receptor, thus clearly targeting the HIV-1 entry process [35].

The antiviral mechanism of Lf appears to be equally complex for the naked viruses, as for the enveloped viruses. Lf has been demonstrated to inhibit replication of rota-, polio- and adenovirus in a dose dependent manner [14, 223, 333]. Apo-Lf was able to bind to the rotavirus particle and prevented both hemaglutination and viral binding to cellular receptors [333]. The effect of iron-saturation of Lf decreased the proteins activity towards rotavirus slightly. A further decrease in activity was also observed with Mg^{2+} or Zn^{2+} saturation of Lf [334]. Antiviral activity towards poliovirus generally required the presence of Lf during the viral adsorption step, though zinc saturated Lf strongly inhibited viral infection when added after viral internalization [223]. Inhibition of adenovirus replication also required addition of Lf before or during the viral adsorption step [14]. Lf activity towards adenovirus infection in HEp2-cells, has been demonstrated to be mediated through the N-terminal half of the protein. The mode of action through competition for viral glycosaminoglycanreceptors on the host cells, and the N-terminal portion or Lfcin alone was sufficient to prevent the viral infection [81]. Further studies have demonstrated that this neutralization of adenovirus was due to direct interaction between the structural viral proteins (III and IIIa) and Lf [276]. Both bLf and hLf inhibits the cytopathic effect of enterovirus 71 (EV71) in human embryonal rhabdomyosarcoma cells. However, ongoing infections were resistant to inhibition, suggesting that the antiviral activity of Lf was excreted at the level of viral adsorption [210]. Complementing experiments have demonstrated that Lf interacts with both the host cell membrane and VP1 protein on the surface of the EV71 particle [393]. Echovirus 6, another member of the enterovirus family can infect green monkey kidney cells, which die as a result of apoptosis after infection. This programmed cell death was also inhibited by Lf [349].

Cellular Uptake of Lactoferrin

Given that Lf is a multifunctional molecule able to interact with numerous cellular and viral targets, its cellular localization could be of great importance for its ability to inhibit infection.

Ji and Mahley [173] have illustrated that mutant chinese hamster ovary (CHO) cells (pgsD-677) lacking heparan sulfate, bound much less Lf, compared to wild type CHO cells, confirming that heparan sulfate was an important molecule for Lf interaction. However, these results also suggested that Lf may bind directly to the low-density-lipoprotein receptor-related protein in the absence of heparan sulfate [173]. This may explain binding of Lf to cell surfaces in the absence of heparan sulfate and other glycosaminoglycan molecules [6]. Low-density-lipoprotein receptor-related protein has also been shown to act as an endocytosis-mediating receptor [147], thus explaining glycosaminoglycan independent internalization of Lf [6] .

Several mammalian cell types and tissues including monocytes [38], lymphocytes [234], liver [235, 288, 422] and the small intestine [181], have been demonstrated to express a specific receptor for Lf (LfR). Cellular uptake of holo-Lf in the small intestine has been linked to the LfR [336], implying that this receptor has a higher affinity for holo- than apo-Lf. This may explain the differing amounts of apo- and holo-Lf found on the surface of Vero cells, even though they have the same affinity for heparan sulfate [6].

Lf also interacts with nucleolin at the cell surface [202]. Though nucleolin mainly are expressed in the nucleus, it is shuttled to the cell surface and back to the nucleus over the cytoskeleton [151]. The interaction between Lf and nucleolin involves binding domains in both the N- and C-terminal lobes of Lf, and occurs in a glycosaminoglycan independent manner [202]. Translocation however is heparan sulfate dependent and the Lf - nucleolin complex follows the recycling / degradation pathway resulting in nuclear localization of Lf [202].

Andersen *et al.* [6] have also demonstrated internalization of hLf at 4°C [6], a temperature at which the endocytic pathway should suffer considerable suppression [376]. The N-terminal nuclear localization signal [271] and heparin-binding domain of Lf [366], G_1RRRR_5 is probably responsible for this type of Lf internalization. Thus internalization of Lf to the nucleus can be blocked by heparin [18], although there is no evidence linking this internalization to heparan sulfate on the cell surface. Energy independent internalization has also been shown in glycosaminoglycan deficient cells [6]. Small angle scattering studies have demonstrated that both lobes of Lf undergo a substantial conformational change as a result of iron binding, consistent with closure of the inter-domain cleft [123]. Variation in the relative amounts of apo- and holo-hLf detected in glycosaminoglycan deficient cells [6] likely indicates that energy independent internalization through the nuclear localization signal is influenced by the secondary structure of Lf.

In conclusion, several internalization processes have been proposed and confirmed for Lf, including both a receptor induced endocytic pathway; for example using low-density-lipoprotein receptor-related protein, LfR or nucleolin, and/or an energy independent entry involving the nuclear localization sequence.

Thus Lf may use different internalization mechanisms, depending on its iron bound state and the experimental conditions.

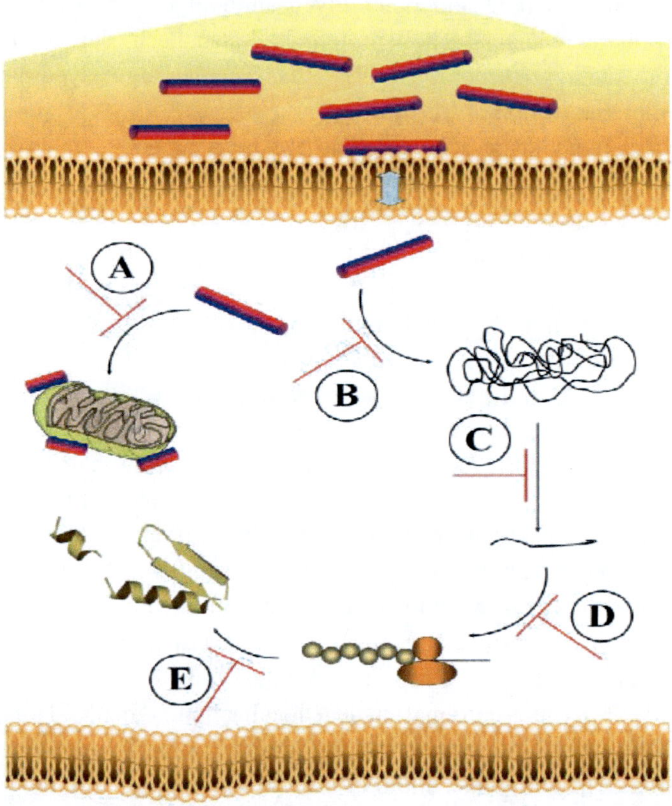

Figure 3. Mechanisms of action of Lf/Lfcin. The cellular membrane is represented as a yellow lipid bilayer with the Lf/Lfcin shown as cylinders where the hydrophilic regions are coloured red and the hydrophobic regions are blue. Extracellular targets for Lf/Lfcin not illustrated on the figure. The translocation mechanism of Lf/Lfcin into the cell is not known. After translocationg the cell membrane Lf/Lfcin interacts with different cellular targets. In tumor cells it has been demonstrated that Lfcin targets the mitochondrial membrane resulting in pore formation, swelling and initially lysis of this eucaritoic organelle (A). Lf/Lfcin has also been shown to inhibit DNA- and RNA synthesis at concentrations lower than their minimal inhibitory concentrations without destabilising the membrane (B and C). Protein synthesis is another possible macromolecular target for Lf/Lfcin (D). Lf has been demonstrated to possess a protease activity and might influence on protein folding and cleavage (E). Figure reprinted and modified from reference [172], with permission from Clinical Microbiology Reviews, Copyright © 2006, American Society for Microbiolog.

Intracellular Targets for Lactoferrin

Little is known about the mechanism behind the immune-stimulating properties of Lf [70, 98, 339]. Intracellular localization of Lf may result in regulation of host cell macromolecular synthesis (figure 3). Several groups have illustrated that Lf are internalized and translocates to the nucleus [6, 202]. It has also been reported that Lf binds a specific DNA sequence [139] and activates the transcription of interleukin (IL)-1β [320]. *In vivo* studies have also demonstrated an increase in serum levels of interleukin-18 and splenocyte production of interferon-γ and interleukin-12 upon orally administration of Lf [386]. These interleukins have the ability to protect the host from infections caused by HSV [350].

Chapter 3

ANTIVIRAL ACTIVITY OF LF DERIVED PEPTIDES

Antimicrobial peptides primarily have antiviral activity towards enveloped RNA and DNA viruses, but lately non-enveloped viruses have also been shown to be susceptible for these peptides. The mode of action is often related to the viral adsorption and entry process [26], or is a result of a direct effect on the viral envelope [1, 292]. However, it appears impossible to predict antiviral activity based primarily on secondary structure of the peptides [172].

In the search for antiviral peptides derived from Lf, it has been demonstrated that two large fragments of bLf, the C-lobe $^{345-689}$ and the N-lobe $^{1-280}$, inhibit HSV-1 infection, while a smaller part of the N-lobe $^{86-258}$ was ineffective [314]. Similarly, the bLf N-lobe $^{86-258}$ and N-lobe $^{324-329}$ were able to inhibit rotavirus infection [334]. However, the most studied fragment of Lf is the highly cationic peptide, Lfcin, isolated from the N-terminal domain. Not surprisingly, due to its net charge and to some extent its amphipathic secondary structure, this peptide has demonstrated high affinity for heparan sulfate [169], an important cell surface molecule involved during many viral infections [240, 326]. Lfcin from different species have been isolated, and tested for its antiviral activity, but most work has been done on LfcinB (bLf$^{17-42}$) [83] and LfcinH (hLf$^{1-49}$) (figure 1 and 2) [155].

LfcinB features a loop region attributable to a disulfide bridge between amino acid residues 19 and 36, a region which is also found in the homologous region of LfcinH (amino acid 20 and 37) [30]. Both LfcinB and LfcinH create a surface-exposed amphipathic α-helical domain in Lf, prior to pepsin digestion [20, 133, 259]. In addition, the larger LfcinH comprises a parallel β-sheet structure. After pepsin cleavage, LfcinB loses its α-helical domain and becomes a distorted antiparallel β-sheet [158], whereas LfcinH retains its α-helical domain but loses its β-sheet [155]. Despite rather diverse structural features both these peptides have demonstrated antiviral activity. LfcinB has been shown to exert antiviral activity against both enveloped e.g. HIV [35], HCMV [7], HSV-1 and HSV-2 [5, 168] and naked viruses e.g. adenovirus [81], feline calicivirus [236], papillomavirus [242], echovirus 6 [275]. LfcinH also has antiviral activity against papillomavirus, HSV-1 and HSV-2, and as observed for other antimicrobial activities, this activity is weaker than for LfcinB towards HSV [5]. Interestingly, LfcinH was found to be a better inhibitor of papillomavirus internalization in comparison with LfcinB [242]. Combinations of Lfcin and acyclovir have also demonstrated synergistic antiviral activity against HSV-1 and HSV-2 [5, 168]. Additionally, acyclovir resistant clinical HSV isolates were also susceptible to inhibition by Lfcin [5].

Structural Requirement for Antiviral Peptides

It has been suggested that the difference in the secondary structure of LfcinB and LfcinH (figure 1) may explain the difference in antiviral activity [5, 168]. However, studies on numerous other antiviral peptides have revealed no direct correlation, neither between the peptide structure and their activity towards a particular virus, nor for the peptides antiviral specificity towards different structural classes of viruses [73, 410]. Extensive amounts of effort have been put into quantitative structural activity relationship studies, in an attempt to identify structural domains required for a peptides antiviral activity. Several groups have looked at the importance of charged and aromatic amino acids, since antiviral peptides are often highly cationic and amphiphilic [73, 168, 342, 410]. The hydrophobic character of different peptides and substitution of D- or L- amino acids have also been investigated [201, 411].

Substitution libraries of LfcinH and LfcinB derived peptides have been constructed and tested for their antiviral activity against HSV-1 and HSV-2 in an attempt to identify primary structure domains contributing to their antiviral activity [169]. N- and C-terminal deletion in LfcinH gave the corresponding human analogue of LfcinB with no detectable antiviral activity [169]. This could be a result of structural changes due to chain length reduction and/or the reduction in net charge from 8.79 to 5.85 at pH 7.0, since antiviral peptides often are described as highly cationic [73, 168, 410]. Relationship between a peptides net charge and its antiviral activity has been reported for both the Lfcin analogues and a set of short α-helical peptides [168-171]. However, the spatial positions of the charged amino acids seem to be more important for antiviral activity than the actual net charge [168, 169].

Several types of charged molecules in the body have been shown to interact through electrostatic interactions with glycosaminoglycan molecules on the host cell surface [56, 82, 150, 159, 185, 211, 216, 262, 268, 273]. Cationic peptide, including several Lfcin analogues have also shown high affinity for heparan sulfate [168, 169] and this affinity increased further if arginine was substituted for lysine [109, 148, 168, 327]. However, even though LfcinH has a higher net positive charge than LfcinB, i.e. 8.79 and 7.84 at pH 7.0, respectively, the two peptides exhibit equal affinity for heparan sulfate, demonstrating that another parameter must influence on the peptide affinity for heparan sulfate [169]. Numerous peptides have been demonstrated to interact with glycosaminoglycan [164] and specific glycosaminoglycan binding domains have been identified in both LfcinH and LfcinB. These domains involve the sequences G_1RRRRS_6 and $R_{28}KVR_{31}$ in LfcinH [220], and the whole sequence of LfcinB [310]. The dispersed positioning of these heparan sulfate binding elements in LfcinH, illustrated that the overall importance depends on how they were presented in the secondary peptide structure.

Aromatic amino acids were known to influence on the secondary folding structure of peptides, due to its hydrophobic potential, thus they may influence heavily on the peptides antiviral activity, like it has been demonstrated for a set of Lfcin derived peptides [168, 169]. The importance of individual amino acids in a peptide has been illustrated by describing the peptide sequence with theoretically derived amino acid descriptors derived by Hellberg *et al.* [141]. These results showed that the terminal amino acids in the LfcinB analogue were of great importance [169]. Although the aromatic nature of these terminal amino acids appears unfavorable, their spatial contribution to the peptide sequence seemed crucial for the antiviral activity [141, 170]. Similar results have been presented by Giansanti *et al.* [118] in a study on shorter peptides derived from bLf and hen ovotransferrin. In this study they concluded that the mixture of hydrophobic and positively charged residues was critical for the peptides antiviral activity, but that these characteristics alone not could explain the antiviral activity of the peptides [118].

The rigid nature of a peptide might also have implication for its antiviral activity, given the structural nature of two of the most potent naturally occurring antiviral peptides found so far, θ-defensin and polyphemusin [342, 411]. The θ-defensins are rather rigid cyclic peptides from old world monkeys [303], while polyphemusin is a β-sheet peptide from the horse shoe crab, where the structure is stabilized by two internal disulfide bridges proven equally crucial for the antiviral activity as the disulfide bridge in LfcinB (figure 1 and 2, table 1 and 2) [7, 169, 342]. A study on a set of short, highly cationic α-helical peptides identify the secondary structural requirements for high anti-HSV activity [168], but the peptides activity could not solely be related to their secondary structure evaluated by circular dichrosim measurements [168]. This is in agreement with results presented by Strøm *et al.* [329, 330], concluding that any peptide helicity present in a solution is non-existent on the cell surface due to flexibility in the peptide structure and a high likelihood of strong interactions with cell surface molecules [329, 330].

The amphipathic structure of LfcinB, with hydrophilic and positively charged residues on opposite sides of the stable β-sheet structure [158], as well as a set of short α-helical peptides [166, 168] are all presumably possessing similar anti-HSV modes of action [168, 169]. This indicates that the peptides are able to interact with their target despite large structural differences. A possible explanation would lie in the observation that these antimicrobial peptides are known to adopt amphipathic conformations that have been proposed to be intrinsic to antiviral activity [172].

Mode of Action of Lfcin Derived Peptides

Blocking of Viral Entry by Heparan Sulphate Interaction

The importance of heparan sulphate for viral infections is well understood in the case of HSV infection. The primary step in HSV infection is attachment of the viral particle to the host cell surface, through interaction with viral glycoprotein C (gC) and /or gB to heparan sulphate [308, 398]. Following the initial attachment to heparan sulphate, other viral glycoproteins interacts with one or several co-receptors on the host cell [325], leading to fusion between the viral envelope and the host cell membrane. Recombinant cells lacking heparan sulphate expression are reduced by 80% in susceptibility to HSV infection [225], however it should be pointed out that the importance of heparan sulphate for viral infection is highly species dependent [240, 326].

Enzymatic removal of cellular heparan sulphate, led to the observation that this molecule has minor influence on HIV attachment to host cells. However, it has been demonstrated that it is of major importance when it came to HIV entry and replication [13]. In contrast, only highly sulphated heparan participated in the entry of HCV [24]. Inhibitors of heparan sulphate, such as heparin, heparinase I treatment, and sodium chlorate, all demonstrated the ability to inhibit HCMV infection in a dose dependent manner [321]. It has even been indicated that naked coxsackievirus B3 made use of a specific modified heparan sulphate molecule for viral entry [418]. One might hypothesize that antimicrobial peptides like Lfcin, with high positive charge, might interact electrostatically with the negatively charge heparan sulphate molecule, thus possess the ability of blocking many different viral infections.

Similar to the specific presentation of charge residues in Lfcin to enable heparan sulphate interaction, a specific pattern of charge and hydrophobic residues are also required in the viral glycoprotein of HSV for interaction with heparan sulphate [355]. The interaction depends highly on the amino acid composition in a sixteen amino acid loop structure in the HSV-1 gC molecule (figure 2). This loop has 87.5% sequence homology with HSV-2 gC [154]. But most interestingly Lfcin creates a similar loop of 16 residues [169] with 87.5% homology to HSV-1 gC when comparing structural groups of amino acid residues rather than identical amino acids, in LfcinB.

It has been demonstrated that cationic peptides can be taken up by cells in an energy independent fashion, which required heparan sulphate [110]. The mechanism was influenced by the arginine content of the peptide [114, 115, 335]. Conversely, transmission electron microscopy studies revealed that LfcinB was able to enter heparan sulphate deficient cells in an energy independent way [6]. This may be explained by a mechanism described by Kim *et al.*, [183] where internalization of arginine rich peptides only partially was inhibited by heparinase III. Another explanation may be the nuclear localization sequence located in LfcinH [271].

Since heparan sulphate works as an attachment receptor for several viruses [240, 326], Lfcin interaction with heparan sulphate might block the viral infection. It has been proposed that Lfcin can block HSV infection by binding to heparan sulphate at the cell surface in a manner similar to Lf [6]. This was supported by the fact that Lfcin has no direct effect on the HSV particle, since allowing Lfcin to interact with the virus did not affect the inhibitory effect of the peptide [6]. Using electron microscopy it has also been demonstrated that LfcinB did not interact directly with the HSV particle, indicating that interactions with HSV glycoprotein's did not occur (Jenssen, H; Unpublished results). The Lfcin peptides also contained specific glycosaminoglycan binding domains [220, 310] and have shown relatively high heparan sulphate affinity [169].

Trybala *et al.* [356] have demonstrated that HSV-2 has higher affinity than HSV-1 for heparan sulphate [356]. HSV-1 has also been shown to be highly dependent on the gC heparan sulphate interaction [358], while HSV-2 gB played a key role in mediating HSV-2 attachment and entry [67]. Thus heparan sulphate blocking affected HSV-1 and HSV-2 interaction differently, explaining why some peptides possessed higher activity towards HSV-1 than HSV-2, and vice versa [168, 169, 171].

A specific HSV entry receptor is a 3-O-sulfated form of heparan sulphate, which interacts with viral gD mediating efficient entry of HSV-1, but not HSV-2 [313, 399]. This receptor is structurally similar to heparan sulphate, except with an additional sulphate in the 3-OH position of the glucosamine residue, thus probably possessing a higher affinity potential for cationic peptides. Lfcin interaction with heparan sulphate molecules containing the 3-O-sulfated binding sites may therefore interfere or block the HSV-1 gD interaction, explaining why several Lfcin analogues show higher antiviral activity against HSV-1 than HSV-2 [169].

Papillomavirus infection of the host cell has been demonstrated to depend on virus interaction with cellular α6β4-integrin complex and heparan sulphate [43, 69, 84, 99, 120, 175, 239, 301, 302, 305, 416]. By use of virus-like particles, it has been demonstrated that LfcinB were able to inhibit host cell infection, and it has been hypothesized that this inhibition was due to interaction and blocking of cellular heparan sulphate [242]. Though, it should be mentioned that not all papillomaviruses required heparan sulphate for host cell infection [270].

Similarly LfcinB have an antiviral activity against HCMV and HIV at the virus-cell interface [7, 35] and this is hypothesized to be related to heparan sulphate binding as well. Binding of HIV to the CD4 surface receptor is known to induce conformational changes in the viral gp120 protein, in the viral envelope, resulting in increased affinity for heparan sulphate. This finding implies that heparan sulphate is important at a later stage of the attachment process of HIV to the host cell membrane [377].

Blocking of Cell-To-Cell Spread

Antiviral effect of cationic peptides may also relate to their ability to inhibit the spread of virus from one cell to a neighboring cell across tight junctions (cell-to-cell spread), or inhibition of syncytia formation. LfcinB like many other peptides [168, 241, 317] possess the ability to inhibit cell-to-cell spread of HSV [6]. Results observed when LfcinB is added after initial attachment of the virus to the cell surface (1 hour at 4°C) or after viral entry (1 hour at 37°C) [6] implies an additional effect of peptides on viral spread from cell-to-cell. A similar ability to reduce cell-to-cell spread has been reported for α-helical peptides [168, 241].

Blocking of Viral Entry by Interaction with Viral Glycoproteins

Antimicrobial peptide interactions with glycoproteins in the viral envelope have been proposed to influence the viral entry process. Additionally, it has been demonstrated that θ-defensin interacts with the HSV-2 glycoprotein B (gB), thus protecting the cells from HSV-2 infection [411]. The polyphemusin analogue T22 inhibited fusion between the HIV envelope and the host cell membrane [247], through specific binding of the viral envelope protein gp120 and the T-cell surface protein CD4 [343]. Lfcin could possess a similar effect, due to structural similarity. Supporting evidence has also confirmed that Lf blocked HIV infection by interfering with CXCR4- and CCR5-receptor interaction. However, these experiments concluded this effect was not due to the N-terminal Lfcin segment in the protein [35].

Intracellular Targets and Host Cell Stimulation

Antimicrobial peptides are able to cross lipid membranes including the plasma and nuclear membranes of host cells, while others are constitutively located as precursors inside host cell vacuoles [6, 137, 200]. Cellular internalization of antimicrobial peptides can eventually influence on host cell antiviral mechanisms by stimulating host cell gene/protein expression [45], or blocking of viral gene/protein expression [384]. By use of transmission electron microscopy, it has been demonstrated that Lfcin translocates intracellularly, in an energy- and heparan sulphate independent manner [6]. A similar mechanism was described by Futaki *et al.* [114, 115, 335], in which the arginine content of the peptides was an important factor, as it is a known feature of the nuclear localization signals. The multiple arginine patches in LfcinH [271] probably contributed to the shuttling of this peptide into the nucleus, where it can bind DNA. Due to the ability of peptides to interact with DNA, [152, 180, 266, 322] one might speculate that Lfcin directly can influence viral nucleic acid synthesis, as has been shown for Lf. Although still controversial, it has been suggested that α-defensin-1 was the soluble $CD8^+$ T-cell antiviral factor with potent activity against HIV [60]. Similar immune activating properties were also hypothesized for Lfcin.

Chapter 4

ANTIBACTERIAL ACTIVITY OF LF

One of the first antimicrobial functions discovered for Lf was its ability to sequester iron from a bacterial pathogen (table 3) [16, 54], thus inhibiting the bacterial growh rate. For a long time it was believed that this was the only antibacterial mode of action of Lf. This was supported by several studies demonstrating that only apo- (iron-free) lactoferrin possessed antibacterial activity, and that this activity was reduced upon iron-saturation [15, 177, 404]. Arnold *et al.* [17] were the first to demonstrate that Lf also were able to kill *Streptocuccus mutans* through an iron-independent mechanism [17]. This activity was later hypothesized to be a result of a direct interaction between Lf and the bacterial cell surface (table 3) [42, 74].

Crystal structure studies of Lf have demonstrated that the protein has large cationic patches on the protein surface [21]. Lf has been demonstrated to interact directly with the anionic lipid A parts of lipopolysaccharide of Gram-negative bacteria [12, 46], primarily through interactions involving the N-terminal regions of Lf, in a domain overlapping the Lfcin region [88, 249, 352, 381]. Interaction between Lf and bacterial lipopolysaccharide, damages the bacterial membrane, alters the outer membrane permeability, and results in a release of lipopolysaccharide [93]. This effect was effectively inhibited by divalent cations like Mg^{2+} and Ca^{2+}, leading Ellison *et al.* to hypothesize that Lf could work as cation chelator like EDTA [94], which also is known to induce lipopolysaccharide release from bacterial membranes [250]. Direct binding of Ca^{2+} by Lf has recently been confirmed, strengthening the cation chelator hypothesis [294], thus also explaining the broad antibacterial spectrum of Lf [380, 390].

Table 3. Biological activity of lactoferrin

Activity	Target	Mode of action	References
		Iron sequestering	[16, 31, 54]
Antibacterial	G-+/- bacteria	Damage bacterial membrane	[93]
		Protease activity – cleave bacterial virulence proteins	[122, 255, 285]
Antiviral	HSV	Targets adsorption / entry – no effect on the viral particle	[6]
	HCMV	Targets adsorption / entry – no effect on the viral particle	[7, 134]
	RS-virus	Unknown	[124]
	Hepatitis B	Targets cellular molecules interfering with viral attachment / entry	[132]
	Hepatitis C	Targets viral envelope protein E1 and E2 – block entry	[160, 161, 412]
	Hepatitis G	Unknown	[160]
	HIV	Targets V3 loop in envelope protein gp120 – block CXCR4- or CCR5-attachment	[35, 134, 284, 337]
	Hantavirus	Targets adsorption / entry (not heparan sulphate) – no effect on the viral particle	[246]
	Rotavirus	Interact with viral particle preventing hemaglutination and attachment to cellular receptors	[333]
	Poliovirus	Target viral adsorption / compete for viral receptor interaction	[223]
	Adenovirus	Target viral adsorption / binds viral protein III and IIIa.	[14, 81, 276]
	Enterovirus (EV71 & Echovirus 6)	Target viral adsorption – binds both cellular receptors and the viral surface protein VP1. Inhibit apoptosis	[210, 349, 393]
	Feline herpes virus -1	Target viral attachment/entry	[25]
	Sindbis virus	Targets adsorption / entry – no effect on the viral particle	[383]
	Semliki Forest virus	Targets adsorption / entry – no effect on the viral particle	[383]
Antifungal	*C. albicans*	Cell wall perturbation	[31, 400]
Antiparasitic	*Pneumocystis carinii*	Iron sequestering	[392]
Antitumor	Several tumor lines	Cytotoxic to the tumor cells	[237]

By damaging the bacterial membrane, Lf is able to increase the antibacterial effect of commercial drugs like rifampicin [93]. More interestingly there is synergy, between Lf, lysozyme and other proteins secreted on the mucosal surface [92, 316]. The proposed mechanism is that Lf interaction with lipoteichoic acid in the membrane of *Staphylococcus epidermidis* result in a decrease in the negative charge in the membrane, allowing lysozyme to reach peptidoglycans buried deeper in the membrane [204].

A more recent discovery is that the N-terminal lobe of Lf possesses a protease activity. By use of protease inhibitors it was suggested that Lf has a serine-protease-like activity, and it has been demonstrated that it is able to degrade IgA1 and Hap, two autotransported proteins from *Haemophilus influenzae*, thus attenuating the bacteria and preventing colonization [285]. Further studies have also reveal that Lf is able to cleave proteins in arginine-rich regions, and that the active sight is situated in the N-terminal lobe [143].

Numerous bacterial strains have developed an ability to infect human cells. When sensing the presence of potential target cells these bacterial strains start secreting virulence proteins from a complex type III secretion system [39, 55, 102, 165, 179]. Lf has the ability to degrade some of these proteins, like two proteins (IpaB and IpaC) secreted by *Shigella*. These proteins normally form a complex in the host cell membrane, and are key components responsible for bacterial-directed phagocytosis, thus their degradation will inhibit bacterial invasion [122, 255]. Similar effects are also observed on enteropathogenic *Escherichia coli* where Lf causes loss and degradation of several type III secretion protein (EspA, EspB and EspC), thus inhibit bacterial virulence, blocking bacterial adherence, and inducing actin polymerization in HEp2 cells [255-257]. It can not be ruled out that Lf also may exhibit a protease activity after internalization into the host cell, thus stimulating different immune mechanisms (figure 4).

Aggregation of bacterial cells and the formation of biofilm are well studied phenomena, especially for *Pseudomonas aeruginosa*, the leading cause of morbidity and mortality in cystic fibrosis patients. By changing the bacterial way and allowing biofilm formation, the bacteria also becomes highly resistant to host cell defense mechanisms and antibiotic treatment [258]. However interestingly, Lf inhibits biofilm formation of *P. aeruginosa* at concentrations lower that those needed to kill the bacteria or prevent its regular growth [315].

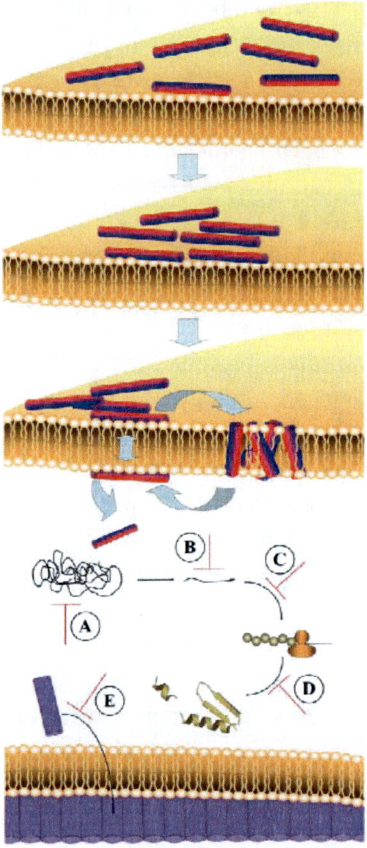

Figure 4. Mechanisms of action of Lfcin. The bacterial membrane is represented as a yellow lipid bilayer with the peptides shown as cylinders where the hydrophilic regions are coloured red and the hydrophobic regions are blue. Cell wall associated peptidoglycan molecules are depicted as purple cylinders. Membrane permeabilisation of Lfcin is illustrated by the aggregate model. In this model Lfcin reorient to span the membrane as an aggregate with micelle-like complexes of peptides and lipids, but without adopting any particular orientation. Other membrane permeabilising models for antimicrobial peptides have been reviewed elsewhere [53, 172], and can not be totally excluded as possible models for Lfcin as well. After translocationg the bactherial cell membrane both Lf and Lfcin has been shown to inhibit DNA- and RNA synthesis at concentrations lower than their minimal inhibitory concentrations without destabilising the membrane (A and B). Protein synthesis is another macromolecular target for Lfcin, which have been shown to decrease the rate of protein synthesis in target bacterial cells quite instantly after exposure to the peptide (C). Lf has been demonstrated to possess a protease activity and might influence on protein folding and cleavage (D). Several antimicrobial peptides have been demonstrated to inhibit cell wall synthesis, but this mechanism has not yet been confirmed for Lfcin (E). Figure reprinted and modified from reference [172], with permission from Clinical Microbiology Reviews, Copyright © 2006, American Society for Microbiolog.

Lf increases the susceptibility of *S. epidermidis* biofilms to lysozyme and vancomycin [205]. The process of biofilm formation for several bacterial strains requires higher levels of iron than is needed for regular growth of the specific bacteria, thus Lf as an iron chelator has been hypothesized to effectively inhibit biofilm formation through iron sequestering [391]. Addition of iron or iron-saturated Lf (holo-Lf) to the media have also demonstrated an induction of both *P. aeruginosa* and *B. cepacia* aggregates evolving into biofilms, thus confirming this hypothesis [36].

The importance of iron for bacterial growth in combination with the iron sequestering ability of Lf [16, 54] have stimulated bacterial strains to develop strategies to overcome iron depletion. Under iron-restricted conditions a number of Gram-negative bacterial pathogens have developed mechanisms for acquiring the iron-ion back from the Lf. The mechanism involved binding of Lf to an Lf-receptor on the bacterial surface. This receptor was composed of two Lf binding proteins, (LbpA and LbpB) [207, 272]. It has been proposed that Lf binding to LbpA results in a conformational change in the C-lobe of Lf resulting in release of iron into the periplasmic compartment where it interacts with iron-binding proteins which transports it further into the cell [87]. *Streptococcus pneumoniae* has specifically been shown to recognize and bind hLf, with a surface receptor homologue to pneumococcal surface protein A, and it was concluded that *S. pneumoniae* may use this receptor to overcome the iron limitation at mucosal surfaces [126]. Similar Lf-receptors have also been identified on the surface of *Helicobacter pylori* [80].

In *Escherichia coli* it has been shown that Lf interacts with two porins OmpF and OmpC, in a mechanism of delivering iron to the bacteria [97]. *Mycoplasma pneumoniae* have a highly specific receptor for recognizing and binding Lf, but not the closely related transferrein [359]. In addition, Lf receptors have also been identified on *Neisseria gonorrhoeae* [9], *Neisseria meningitides* [283] and on non-encapsulated *Haemophilus influenzae* [379].

Chapter 5

ANTIBACTERIAL ACTIVITY OF LFCIN

Lf derived peptides with antibacterial activity, and especially Lfcin have been studies extensively over the past decades [100]. It is well understood that regardless of their actual origin and mode of action, all types of antibacterial cationic peptides must interact with the bacterial cytoplasmic membrane [131]. The physical forces behind antibacterial activity have been defined in detail (see [75, 130, 131] for overviews) and it include; net positive charge which enhance the interaction with anionic lipids and other bacterial targets, hydrophobicity allows insertion of the peptide into the bacterial membrane, and flexibility permitting the peptide to transition from its solution conformation to its membrane interacting conformation. Each of these characteristics can vary substantially over a particular range, but are essential for the peptides function as antimicrobial agents and allows them to interact with bacterial membranes, which is critical to them exerting antimicrobial effects.

The way antimicrobial peptides interact with the prokaryotic cell membrane has been extensively investigated [11, 96, 232, 319]. Due to the fact that most antimicrobial peptides are cationic at physiological pH, they are prone to interact quite unspecifically through electrostatic interactions, with negatively charged molecules in the bacterial cell membrane. In Gram-negative bacteria these negatively charged molecules are lipopolysaccharide while in Gram-positive bacteria these molecules are lipoteichoic acid and/or teichoic acid. Experiments have demonstrated that Lfcin can bind both lipopolysaccharide and teichoic acid [62, 382]. Several Lfcin homologues from different species e.g. human (H), caprine (C), murine (M), procine (P) and bovine (B) have been investigated for their antibacterial activity (table 2). Bovine Lfcin (LfcinB) has been reported to posses a bactericidal activity towards a wide variety of both Gram-negative and -

positive bacteria, meaning that it prevents infection by killing these microorganisms (table 4) [29, 83, 312, 404]. Human Lfcin (LfcinH) on the other hand has only bacteriostatic activity towards a panel of Gram-negative and -positive bacteria, meaning that it is capable of inhibiting the growth or reproduction of the bacteria, but not kill it (table 4) [29, 83, 404]. A 20 amino acid residue segment of porcine Lfcin (LfcinP) corresponding to pLf $^{18-37}$ has been reported to display antimicrobial activity against *E. coli, S. aureus* and *C. albicans*. The peptide was four times more active than LfcinH but slightly less active than LfcinB [64]. In conclusion, LfcinB has superior bactericidal activity compared to the other Lfcin peptides [328, 381]. Gram-positive bacteria have also been shown more susceptible to Lfcin than Gram-negative bacteria, probably due to the lack of an outer membrane [363].

However the results also demonstrate that despite very different secondary peptide structure, both LfcinB and LfcinH are able to excrete antibacterial activity. This is consistent with antibacterial measurements for other antimicrobial peptides, concluding that antibacterial activity and spectrum of a peptide not can be extrapolated from the peptides secondary structure [106, 172]. In general the antibacterial activity of cationic peptides seems largely to be affected by amphipathic and amphiphilic patches in their folded structure and by regions with high concentration of positively charged residues [281].

The antibacterial activity of Lfcin has primarily been ascribed to its net charge, giving it an ability to initiate electrostatic interactions with the pathogen [331]. Murine Lfcin (LfcinM) which contains two glutamic acid residues, lacks detectable antibacterial activity (table 1 and 2) [381]. Amidation of the C-terminal end of the peptides have also been demonstrated to increase their activity [331]. However, modulation of the antibacterial activity of cationic peptide through alteration of their hyrdophobicity or net charge may also alter the selectivity between the desired bacterial target and the host cell [197, 419]. Similarly, incorporation of charged residues above a certain maximum (varying from peptide to peptide) does not lead to an increase in activity [75]. Thus this balance of charge and hydrophobicity can be delicate and must be empirically determined for each series of peptides.

Quantitative structure activity relation studies on LfcinB have revealed that the two tryptophan residues are central for the peptides antibacterial activity [328]. These hydrophobic residues interact with the lipophilic part of the membrane, stabilizing the charge-charge interaction between the peptide and the lipid head groups. Optimization studies introducing several tryptophan residues in different positions have indicated that more tryptophan residues may enhance the membrane thinning effect [328]. These results correlate with the fact that LfcinH,

LfcinM and LfcinC which only contain one tryptophan in the homologue region of LfcinB possesses a weak or no antibacterial activity [381]. The advantage of bulky side chains for stable membrane interaction and disruption may also explain the favoring of arginine before lysine as the prime amino acid residue for charge interaction [178].

Table 4. Biological activity of lactoferricin

Activity	Target	Mode of action	References
Antibacterial	G-+/- bacteria	Depolarization of cytoplasmic membrane	[29, 83, 312]
		Inhibition of DNA, RNA and protein synthesis	[363, 404]
Antiviral	HCMV	Activity at virus-cell interface	[7]
	HIV	Unknown	
	HSV	Blocks heparan sulphate, but a secondary effect has also been indicated.	[5, 169]
	Papilloma virus	Activity at virus-cell interface	[242]
Antifungal	*C. albicans*	Cell wall damage	[31, 370]
Antitumor	Several tumor lines	Depolarization of the mitochondrial membrane	[89]

In addition to anchoring the peptides in the bacterial membrane, the bulky side chains also appears to play an important roll for the peptides selectivity towards different types of bacteria, where bulky side chains appear to be more important for *S. aureus* activity than for *E. coli* activity [136]. Smaller deletion peptides of LfcinB have also been investigated, and the results demonstrate that an amidated hexamer section (RRWRWR-NH_2) of LfcinB retains antibacterial activity comparable to the native LfcinB [352]. The results, demonstrating that shorter Lfcin derivatives retain most of the antibacterial activity, correlate with the results demonstrating that the disulfide bridge in LfcinB have very little effect on the peptides antibacterial activity [32, 149].

ANTIBACTERIAL MODE OF ACTION OF LFCIN

It was originally proposed that permeabilization of the bacterial cell membrane was the sole mode of action of antibacterial peptides [250]. Today there is an increasing body of evidence, however, indicating that some antimicrobial peptides exert their effects through alternative modes of action, or in fact may act upon multiple bacterial cell targets. Regardless of their precise mode of action, the activities of antibacterial peptides are almost universally dependent upon interaction with the bacterial cell membrane [131]. In addition, while most cationic antibacterial peptides studied so far have been characterized as membrane-permeabilizing, it should be noted that virtually any cationic amphiphilic peptide will cause membrane perturbation in model systems if a high enough concentration is applied [269, 421]. Model membrane systems using artificial salt and pH conditions, could possibly also mask alternative mechanisms or overestimate the membrane permeabilizing activity.

However, following membrane interaction, Lfcin crosses the outer lipid layer of the bacteria to interact with its cytoplasmic membrane, in a mechanism termed the aggregate model, involving self-promoted uptake (figure 4) [127, 128, 378, 397]. The aggregate model can explain both membrane permeabilization whereby informal channels are formed in a variety of sizes for variable lengths of time [397], as well as translocation across the bilayer that is known to occur for several peptides [282]. Three other models of the interaction of antimicrobial peptide with bacterial cell membranes are; the toroidal pore model [125, 145, 231, 406], the barrel-stave model [86, 140, 324, 421] and the carpet model [280, 403]. However, these models generally explain the pore-forming ability of α-helical antibacterial peptides and have never been demonstrated for β-sheet peptides such as LfcinB [96, 131, 269, 421]. Studies with fragments of LfcinH have demonstrated that these peptides can self-associate in the presence of lipopolysaccharide, forming a tightly packed aggregate [61]. It has been confirmed that Lfcin acts relatively slow on the bacteria, resulting in collapse of the membrane potential, membrane integrity and cell lysis [62]. It has also been demonstrated that Lfcin compromises the membrane permeability, causing a depolarization of the bacterial cytoplamic membrane and loss of pH gradient [2]. Nuclear magnetic resonance spectroscopy studies of membrane interactions with LfcinB derived peptides have also suggested that alterations in the peptide sequence can result in deeper embedding of the tryptophan residues in the inner membrane, resulting in more active peptides [248]. Insertion of peptides or aggregates of peptides into the membrane has also been hypothesized to be the reason for formation of membrane blebs on the surface of certain bacterial cells exposed to LfcinB [312, 404]. Any aggregate of peptides has the potential to disrupt the outer membrane structure, through interactions with both hydrophobic and hydrophilic faces of the membrane, resulting in disruption of the fluidity of the membrane, permitting translocation of peptides and thus permitting access to other potentially lethal targets [61].

It is well established that several antimicrobial peptides do not cause membrane permeabilization at the minimal effective concentration, yet still result in bacterial death. A growing number of peptides translocate to the membrane and accumulate at intracellular targets. Novel modes of action include inhibition of nucleic acid synthesis, protein synthesis, enzymatic activity and cell wall synthesis (figure 4) [53]. Electron microscopy studies demonstrate that LfcinB quite easily enters into both Gram-positive and Gram-negative bacteria [137, 297, 298], thus it is debated whether the depolarization of the bacterial membrane is a result of alteration of metabolic pathways in the bacteria in stead of Lfcin interaction with the bacterial membrane [137]. A number of potential antibacterial targets are in reach after internalization of Lfcin. Exposure of the Gram-positive bacterium, *Bacillus subtilis*, to sub-lethal concentrations of LfcinB inhibit DNA, RNA and protein synthesis (figure 4) [363]. Similar modes of action for Gram-negative bacteria [363], though this picture is a bit more complex, involve a multi-phase mode of action, similar to what has been demonstrated for other cationic antimicrobial peptides [58]. Though β-sheets like LfcinB traverse the bacterial membrane much easier than α-helical and random coil peptides, several other non β-sheet peptides also translocate across the lipid bilayer and inhibit the macromolecular synthesis [41, 107, 156, 203, 266, 269, 332].

Chapter 6

ANTIFUNGAL ACTIVITY OF LF

Candida is looked upon as a commencal organism in healthy individuals, and can colonize mucosal surfaces. There is equilibrium between the host and the growth of *Candida*, which is controlled by several nonspecific factors, e.g. immunoglobulin A, lysozyme and histatins, secreted on mucosal surface [264, 278]. Lf is also secreted on mucosal surfaces and has demonstrated antifungal activity against *Candida* [385]. The activity of bLf against *Candida* varies considerably from species to species. A study on six different stains shows the following susceptibility: *C. tropicalis* > *C. krusei* > *C. albicans* > *C. guilliermondii* > *C. parapsilosis* > *C. glabrata*, the latter being the most resistant. In this study the antifungal mode of action of Lf is also proposed to be due to cell wall perturbation, confirmed by cryo-scanning electron microscopy revealed drastic changes in the cell wall, resulting in surface blebs, swelling and cell collapse [400]. Similar cell wall damages due to hLf and bLf exposure are reported by Nikawa *et al.* [252, 253]. Candidacidal activity of hLf is due to direct interactions between the protein and the fungal cell surface, rather than iron sequestering [365].

Recent studies have also indicated that the antifungal activity of Lf can be regulated by the metabolic state of the fungus. These experiments demonstrated that the fungicidal activity of Lf was significantly reduced under anaerobic growth conditions and with addition of mitochondrial inhibitors. The fungicidal activity was also inhibited by low extracellular concentrations of Na^+, K^+, Ca^{2+} and Mg^{2+} [375].

The antifungal activity of Lf has also been reported to be considerably lower than the activity of commercially available antifungal drugs. However, combined use of Lf and several commercial drugs, e.g. clotrimazole, fluconazole, amphotericin B and 5-fluorocytosine, have demonstrated, potential additive and synergistic activity [194, 385]. It has also been indicated that Lf can mediated its antifungal activity through stimulation of host cell immune mechanisms both *in vitro* and *in vivo* [402].

Chapter 7

ANTIFUNGAL ACTIVITY OF LFCIN

The fungal cell wall consists primarily of polysaccharides like β1-3 glucans or chitin that do not have their counterpart in humans [121]. β1-3 glucan have no charge [290] while chitin is highly positively charged [208], thus hypothetically chitin would be repulsive to cationic peptides. However, the antifungal mode of action of cationic peptides was first described as involving either fungal cell lysis as a result of direct interaction between the peptides and the fungal membrane or interference with fungal cell wall synthesis [79]. It should also be mentioned that peptides with primarily antifungal activity, tend to be relatively rich in polar and neutral amino acids, suggesting a unique structure-activity relationship for this type of peptides compared to other antimicrobial peptides [216].

Lfcin appears to possess multiple antifungal mode of action, where the initial effect of the peptide is on the plasma membrane. Direct interaction between LfcinB and the *Candida* cell membrane results in disruption of the fungal membrane [31, 370]. The direct interaction of both LfcinB and LfcinH has also been confirmed to alter the proton gradient across the fungal membrane [215]. A secondary mode of action is an intracellular effect, where parts of the cytoplasmic material have been demonstrated to aggregate as a result of Lfcin exposure. Lfcin also resulted in up-regulation of adenosine 5'-triphosphate (ATP) synthesis, leading to secretion of ATP to extracellular compartments [215, 362]. Extracellular ATP can then work as a cytotoxic mediator by binding to purinergic receptors in the fungal membrane leading to cell death [190, 191]. It has also been suggested that formation of reactive oxygen species was involved in the fungicidal mechanism of histatin 5 and Lfcin-derived peptides [142, 214].

An immunomodulatory activity has also been observed for Lfcin. In a assay using several deletion peptides from the N-terminal part of Lf, a deca-peptide

(FKCRRWQWRM) was able to up-regulate *Candida* cell killing by activation of polymorphonuclear leukocytes, increasing their generation of superoxide, protein kinase C- and p38 MAPK activity [362], has also been proven important in control and evasion of *Candida* infections in a mouse model [195].

Viejo-Diaz *et al.* [374] have identified two novel hLf-derived peptides with different anti-*Candida* activities, but quite high sequence homology with the sequence of another antifungal peptide, brevinin-1Sa [372, 374]. Structure activity relationship studies on three synthetic LfcinB $^{17\text{-}30}$ -derived peptides revealed a significant positive correlation between the pI values of peptides and their candicidal activity [251]. So in conclusion, no conserved sequences are evident for the antifungal peptides, though several have been demonstrated to possess specific biochemical characteristics, such as chitin- [112, 153] or heparin-binding abilities [10, 310]. There is a direct correlation between the peptides ability to form complexes with lipid mixtures and their antifungal activity [212].

LfcinB in combination with clotrimazole have also shown to be synergistic by checkerboard analysis, suggesting that Lf-derived peptides may function co-operatively with azole antifungal agents against *C. albicans* [385].

Chapter 8

ANTIPARASITIC ACTIVITY OF LF

The antiparasitic activity of Lf is not investigated in great detail. However, so far it has been suggested that Lf possesses antiparasitic activity towards *Pneumocystis carinii* through iron sequestering [392]. Interestingly, some parasites have developed ways to counteract the iron sequestering process of Lf. In studies with *Tritrichomonas foetus*, grown under iron restrictions, Lf demonstrated the ability to enhance the growth of the parasite. Lf was also taken up and released from the parasite in an energy dependent mechanism [338].

Plasmodium spp. invasion of cultured cells require that the pathogen protein circumsporazoite recognizes and binds to host cell heparan sulfate. Lf is known to interact strongly with heparan sulfate [169], thus it has been suggested that the anti-plasmodulium activity of Lf is a result of blocking of this receptor [318]. The circumsporazoite protein from *Plasmodium berghei* has also been demonstrated to bind to low low-density-lipoprotein receptor-related protein. However, *P. berghei* invasion of heparan sulfate deficient cells were effectively inhibited with Lf, suggesting that Lf also might bind and block parasite interaction with the low-density-lipoprotein receptor-related protein [306]. Lf also works with additive or synergistic activity with clinically used antiparasitic compounds [68].

Chapter 9

ANTIPARASITIC ACTIVITY OF LFCIN

Magainin 2 was one of the first antimicrobial peptides demonstrated to display antiprotozoan activity, leading to swelling and eventual bursting of *Paramecium caudatum* [417]. Membrane disruption through pore formation, or via direct interaction with the lipid bilayer have later been demonstrated for other peptides [267]. However, little is known about the antiparasitic mode of action of Lfcin. Though it has been demonstrated that Lfcin exerts an antimicrobial activity against a range of protozoa [346, 361].

Studies with sporozoites of *Toxoplasma gondii* and *Eimeria stiedai* have demonstrated that pretreatment of the sporozoites with Lfcin, prior to inoculation into mice, increased the survival rate of the mice [263]. It also seems likely that antiprotozoan activity may be dependent on fundamentally different peptide motifs to those required for bacterial, viral and fungal activity [172].

Chapter 10

ANTITUMOR ACTIVITY OF LF

There is a profound difference between normal healthy cell and tumor cell surfaces, in that tumor cells have a higher content of negatively charged molecules, i.e. phosphatidylserine, lipoproteins, O-glycocylated mucines and sialic acid, on their outer leaflet, relative to normal eukaryotic cells [57, 243, 286, 364, 394, 425]. This difference can explain why Lf can mediate a cytotoxic activity towards oral squamous cell carcinoma, though similar concentrations have no toxic effect on healthy cells [237].

Recombinant human and murine Lf has been demonstrated to inhibit tumor growth of both squamous cell carcinoma and fibrosarcoma in an *in vivo* murine model. Inhibition of growth by more than 50% could be observed after administration of Lf directly into the tumors. Interestingly there was a significant effect of Lf in immunocompetent mice, indicating that immune-modulation might be playing a very important role in the antitumor mode of action of Lf [395]. The effect of Lf on inhibition of tumor metastasis in L51778Y-ML25 cells in another mouse model, demonstrated that this activity was dependent on bLf being administered in its apo form and that iron saturation resulted in loss of activity. It was further shown that apo-hLf had no activity [415].

In addition to possess an antitumor activity, Lf has also been demonstrated to stimulate proliferation in normal cells. Lf and human neutrophil peptide-1 have both demonstrated the ability to mediate cytotoxicity towards oral squamous cell carcinoma. At high concentrations similar cytotoxicity effects can be observed towards normal oral keratinocytes. However, when combining Lf and human neutrophil peptide-1 at concentrations non-toxic for the normal oral keratinocytes, a different effect was observed. In the normal cells, proliferation was stimulated, while in squamous carcinoma cells an induction of cell death was observed, indicating an important co-operative role for Lf with other antimicrobial host defense peptides [237].

Chapter 11

ANTITUMOR ACTIVITY OF LFCIN

The specific charge difference in the cell membrane of tumor cells and healthy cells can clearly explain why numerous antimicrobial peptides, including LfcinB, have been shown to exert a selective cytotoxic activity towards cancer cells over normal cells [23, 65, 72, 90, 174, 260, 364, 407, 408]. In addition, different modes of action of antimicrobial peptides have been demonstrated towards different cancer cells. Both receptor-mediated and receptor-independent internalization of antimicrobial peptides into the eukaryotic cells have been demonstrated to result in disruption of the mitochondrial membrane, followed by release of apoptogenic factors i.e. cytocrome c [192], thus resulting in induction of apoptosis [91, 218]. Classical antimicrobial peptides like magainin, buforin and BMAP-28 spontaneously translocate into the cytoplasm, resulting in depolarization of the inner mitochondrial membranes [291, 341].

The mechanism, by which the peptides are able to kill the tumor cells but not healthy cells, appears to be rather general, given that e.g. Meth A fibrosarcoma, B16F10 melanoma and C26 colon carcinoma cells lines all are susceptible to inhibition by Lfcin [90]. By comparing the cytotoxic activity of LfcinB against neuroblastoma cell lines and healthy human fibroblasts (MRC-5), an 11-fold higher activity has been shown towards the neuroblastoma cells [89]. Interestingly this cytotoxic effect was totally abolished for the linear homologue of LfcinB, implying that the rigid structure of LfcinB might be crucial for its activity [89].

Since Lfcin translocates spontaneously into healthy cells [6], a similar mechanism has been anticipated and later proven for tumor cells [89]. Once internalized, LfcinB has been demonstrated to result in induction of apoptosis in human leukemic (THP-1) and carcinoma cell lines *in vitro* [217, 413, 415], while untransformed lymphocytes, fibroblasts and endothelial cells were not affected.

The apoptosis induced by LfcinB in human THP-1 cells was blocked by addition of antioxidants. In addition, LfcinB treatment of the cells revealed a dose dependent increase in the levels of intracellular reactive oxygen species, suggesting that the apoptosis induced activity was regulated through pathways regulating intracellular reactive oxygen species [413]. The level of reactive oxygen species has also been shown to increase in response to LfcinB treatment in Jurakt T leukemia cells. In these cells, it was demonstrated that LfcinB resulted in mitochondrial swelling and release of cytocrome c (figure 3) [217]. The effect on the mitochondria is consistent with other results gained by use of fluorescently labeled LfcinB by Eliassen *et al.* [89]. In this study, LfcinB translocated to mitochondrial compartments resulting in a punctuated red fluorescence pattern in JC-1-labled Kelly cells. Changes in the mitochondrial membrane potential were further demonstrated by flow cytometry, suggesting that the mitochondria are one of the main targets for LfcinB (figure 3) [89]. By use of selective caspase inhibitors it has been demonstrated that LfcinB induces caspase-dependent apoptosis in human leukemia- and carcinoma cell lines [217]. It is also known that LfcinB causes DNA fragmentation and morphological changes consistent with apoptosis in MDA-MB-435 breast cancer cells [113].

A small library of LfcinB derived peptides has been constructed and quantitative structure activity relationship analysis has been performed to elucidate the structural basis for antitumor activity of Lf-derived peptides. The results demonstrated a strong correlation between antitumor activity and the peptides net positive charge. By increasing the hydrophobicity of the peptides, their antitumor activity could also be increased even further. By shortening the peptide sequences, it was demonstrated that the overall size of the peptide seemed to play a crucial roll for maintaining the antitumor activity [409]. Similar results have been observed for antiviral peptides [169], while antibacterial activity seems to be less influenced of the peptides chain length [352].

LfcinB and other antimicrobial peptides have also demonstrated an activity against solid tumors, e.g. LfcinB has an ability to reduce the size of solid Meth A tumors. [90]. In *in vitro* experiments, LfcinB exposure resulted in swelling and bursting of Meth A cells, a mechanism which could be associated with necrosis [90]. LfcinB also inhibits metastasis, the spread of the cancer from its primary site to other places in the body, in both a murine melanoma and lymphoma model [414, 415].

Chapter 12

NOVEL APPLICATIONS AND CLINICAL USE OF LF AND LF-DERIVED PEPTIDES

Lf has for a long time been isolated from whey, a by-product (once considered as waste) from cheese and curd manufacturing. However, the clinical relevance of using bLf instead of hLf, as a supplement in the human diet has been debated. Thus, considerable amount of work has been put in to producing recombinant human Lf (r-hLf).

RECOMBINANT LF AND LFCIN

Production of r-hLf was first reported in 1994, when Platenburg *et al.* [277] demonstrated expression of hLf in the milk of transgenic mice [277]. Large scale production was later reported in tobacco plants [296] and in the milk of a transgenic cow [367]. However, concerns were raised regarding the risk of bovine pathogens from transgenic cattle. Thus fermentation technology was applied and today Agennix (USA) is producing large quantities of pharmaceutical-grade r-hLf in *Aspergillus* [4]. R-pLf has also successfully been produced with fermentation technology in the methylotropic yeast *Pichia pastoris*, resulting in clones expressing r-pLf at levels constituting 30% of total protein. Though most of the recombinant protein was located in cell cytoplasm, about 10% of the protein was secreted out into the culture supernatant during a 72 hours production cycle. The antibacterial activity of r-pLf was demonstrated to be similar to pLf isolated from porcine milk [63]. Constitutive expression of full length hLf in rice plants under control of the cauliflower mosaic virus 35S promoter, demonstrated that the r-hLf could confer disease resistance in plants, challenged with *Burkholderia plantarii*. A similar effect should be observed with transgenic expression of the N-lobe of hLf, and glycosylation with plant-type oligosaccharide chains did not appear to have any effect on the proteins antimicrobial activity [340].

Similarly, recombinant LfcinB has successfully been produced, utilizing E. coli and a pGEX-4T-2 vector encoding LfcinB as a fusion protein GST-Th-LfcinB [103]. LfcinB was cleaved from the fusion protein by use of thrombine, a protease recognizing a six amino acid cleavage site (-Leu-Val-Pro-Arg-Gly-Ser-) and cleaving specifically the peptide bound between arginine and glycine. Thus the produced LfcinB has an N-terminal Gly-Ser-tail, and the importance of this element has not explored fully in respect to the peptides antimicrobial activity.

CLINICAL APPLICATIONS

As the problem of emergence of bacterial resistance to current antibiotic drugs continues to grow, there has been considerable interest in the development of antimicrobial peptides as a novel therapeutic approach to treat infections as well. Resistance problems for fungal treatment and a very limited number of treatment alternatives for several viral diseases has fuelled this research even more, and the current status has been reviewed elsewhere [172, 226, 420].

The benefit of Lf treatment has been well documented for several viral diseases; e.g. in a rat CMV model [28], in a hantavirus infection model in suckling mice [245] and a influenza (A/PR/8/34 H1N1) model with BALB/c mice [311]. Lf has also been used *in vivo* in the treatment of human hepatitis C virus infections [261, 344]. Though the effect on the HCV disease reduction still is debated, a mechanism of therapeutic action has been suggested [163, 188]. Oral administration of Lf in children vertically infected with HIV-1 has also been evaluated in combination with antiretroviral therapy. The results demonstrated that the combination of Lf and antiretroviral therapy gave an improvement in the $CD4^+$ cell count, compared to antiretroviral therapy treatment alone [424]. The clinical relevance of Lf in HIV infected individuals has also been studied after intravenous administration of the protein. The results demonstrated that Lf rapidly was cleared from the plasma; however immunohistochemical analysis revealed high levels of hLf in endothelial cells in the liver. Small amounts of hLf were also detected in the lymphatic system. This clearly demonstrates that hLf may reach target cells and body compartments crucial for both HCMV and HIV replication [27].

In vivo effects have also been demonstrated for Lf derived peptides. AM-Pharma Holding BV (Netherland) have announced that they have completed phase I clinical trials with an 11-mer peptide derived from the N-terminus of hLf (hLF $^{1-11}$) (table 2). This peptide has been proven efficacious in animal models of osteomyelitis [100] but also other bacterial infections [249]. By use of hLf $^{1-11}$ AM-Pharma seeks to target the prevention of infections in patients undergoing stem cell transplantation. Postoperative infections in these patients are quite severe, and often mortal. Subsequently, they have also suggested that they will develop this compound as a systemic antifungal drug.

Another novel application for Lf has recently been demonstrated by Oyane *et al.* [265] in an attempt to limit the problem with bacterial infections related to percutaneous implants. By use of polymer technology they demonstrated that it was possible to create ethylene-vinyl alcohol copolymer with immobilized Lf on its surface. The composite material demonstrated antibacterial activity against *E. coli* and *S. aureus*. Thus percutaneous devices that are highly resistant to bacterial infection may be developed from this type of composite material in the future [265].

Immune Modulation

Different dietary products directed for children are in parts of the world often supplemented with Lf. The health benefit of this is disputed, however, increasing amount of evidence have demonstrated that Lf supplement may work beneficially on the immune flora. Peptides with antimicrobial activity (Lfcin) are in addition released upon pepsin digestion, and might contribute further to the host defense against microbial attack under *in vivo* conditions [353]. Orally administered bLf has been documented to increases natural killer cell populations in peripheral blood and spleen in a dose dependent manner, in addition to increase interferon-γ production. BLf also increased natural killer cell migration and increased interleukin levels. Collectively, these results demonstrate that oral administration of bLf stimulates intestinal associated immune functions including production of interleukin-18 and type I interferons [193]. Lf induced interferon-α expression in neuroblastoma SK-N-SK cells in addition to inhibiting interleukin-6 production induced by enterovirus 71 [393]. In a BALB/c mouse model, a positive correlation exsisted between the antiviral activity of Lf against influenza A virus and the serum levels of interleukin-6 and other pro-inflammatory cytokine [311].

Chapter 13

CONCLUSION

Lf has an antibacterial activity towards a spectrum of different pathogens, through iron sequestering, membrane destabilization and intracellular bacterial suppression. The antiviral activity of Lf is primarily related to inhibition of viral host cell interaction through blocking of host cell heparan sulfate or interaction with viral surface proteins. The antifungal effect of Lf is predominantly linked to iron sequestering and destabilization of the fungal membrane. Similar membrane activity is observed towards tumor cells. The antiparasitic activity of Lf appears to rely on different mechanisms than for the other microbial activities.

Comparably, Lfcin possesses strong antibacterial and antifungal activity, due to membrane permeabilization. The antiviral activity appears to be quite similar as for the entire protein, though cell surface localization of Lfcin is not required for antiviral activity, indicating a dual antiviral mode of action. The antiparasitic activity is clearly dependent on other structural parameters that the other antimicrobial activities, clearly underlining separate modes of action. The antitumor activity of Lfcin is dependent on internalization of the peptide, where the main target appears to be the mitochondrial membrane.

In general the antimicrobial mode of action of Lf and Lfcin is strongly dependant on the experimental conditions, thus demonstrating their tremendous ability to exercise a diverse range of antimicrobial effects. Increasing insight into the diverse immunomodulatory activities of both Lf and Lfcin are the most recent characterized property and makes them very interesting candidates for new supplementing therapeutics.

Acknowledgment

The author greatly acknowledge Dr. Danna Hargett for valuable suggestions and linguistic assistance.

REFERENCES

[1] Aboudy, Y., E. Mendelson, I. Shalit, R. Bessalle, and M. Fridkin. 1994. Activity of two synthetic amphiphilic peptides and magainin-2 against herpes simplex virus types 1 and 2. *Int J Pept Protein Res* 43:573-82.

[2] Aguilera, O., H. Ostolaza, L. M. Quiros, and J. F. Fierro. 1999. Permeabilizing action of an antimicrobial lactoferricin-derived peptide on bacterial and artificial membranes. *FEBS Lett* 462:273-7.

[3] Almaas, H., H. Holm, T. Langsrud, R. Flengsrud, and G. E. Vegarud. 2006. In vitro studies of the digestion of caprine whey proteins by human gastric and duodenal juice and the effects on selected microorganisms. *Br J Nutr* 96:562-9.

[4] Andersen, J. H. 2004. Technology evaluation: rh lactoferrin, Agennix. *Curr Opin Mol Ther* 6:344-9.

[5] Andersen, J. H., H. Jenssen, and T. J. Gutteberg. 2003. Lactoferrin and lactoferricin inhibit Herpes simplex 1 and 2 infection and exhibit synergy when combined with acyclovir. *Antiviral Res* 58:209-15.

[6] Andersen, J. H., H. Jenssen, K. Sandvik, and T. J. Gutteberg. 2004. Anti-HSV activity of lactoferrin and lactoferricin is dependent on the presence of heparan sulphate at the cell surface. *J Med Virol* 74:262-71.

[7] Andersen, J. H., S. A. Osbakk, L. H. Vorland, T. Traavik, and T. J. Gutteberg. 2001. Lactoferrin and cyclic lactoferricin inhibit the entry of human cytomegalovirus into human fibroblasts. *Antiviral Res* 51:141-9.

[8] Anderson, B. F., H. M. Baker, E. J. Dodson, G. E. Norris, S. V. Rumball, J. M. Waters, and E. N. Baker. 1987. Structure of human lactoferrin at 3.2-A resolution. *Proc Natl Acad Sci U S A* 84:1769-73.

[9] Anderson, J. E., M. M. Hobbs, G. D. Biswas, and P. F. Sparling. 2003. Opposing selective forces for expression of the gonococcal lactoferrin receptor. *Mol Microbiol* 48:1325-37.

[10] Andersson, E., V. Rydengard, A. Sonesson, M. Morgelin, L. Bjorck, and A. Schmidtchen. 2004. Antimicrobial activities of heparin-binding peptides. *Eur J Biochem* 271:1219-26.

[11] Andreu, D., and L. Rivas. 1998. Animal antimicrobial peptides: an overview. *Biopolymers* 47:415-33.

[12] Appelmelk, B. J., Y. Q. An, M. Geerts, B. G. Thijs, H. A. de Boer, D. M. MacLaren, J. de Graaff, and J. H. Nuijens. 1994. Lactoferrin is a lipid A-binding protein. *Infect Immun* 62:2628-32.

[13] Argyris, E. G., E. Acheampong, G. Nunnari, M. Mukhtar, K. J. Williams, and R. J. Pomerantz. 2003. Human immunodeficiency virus type 1 enters primary human brain microvascular endothelial cells by a mechanism involving cell surface proteoglycans independent of lipid rafts. *J Virol* 77:12140-51.

[14] Arnold, D., A. M. Di Biase, M. Marchetti, A. Pietrantoni, P. Valenti, L. Seganti, and F. Superti. 2002. Antiadenovirus activity of milk proteins: lactoferrin prevents viral infection. *Antiviral Res* 53:153-8.

[15] Arnold, R. R., M. Brewer, and J. J. Gauthier. 1980. Bactericidal activity of human lactoferrin: sensitivity of a variety of microorganisms. *Infect Immun* 28:893-8.

[16] Arnold, R. R., M. F. Cole, and J. R. McGhee. 1977. A bactericidal effect for human lactoferrin. *Science* 197:263-5.

[17] Arnold, R. R., J. E. Russell, W. J. Champion, and J. J. Gauthier. 1981. Bactericidal activity of human lactoferrin: influence of physical conditions and metabolic state of the target microorganism. *Infect Immun* 32:655-60.

[18] Ashida, K., H. Sasaki, Y. A. Suzuki, and B. Lonnerdal. 2004. Cellular internalization of lactoferrin in intestinal epithelial cells. *Biometals* 17:311-5.

[19] Baggiolini, M., C. De Duve, P. L. Masson, and J. F. Heremans. 1970. Association of lactoferrin with specific granules in rabbit heterophil leukocytes. *J Exp Med* 131:559-70.

[20] Baker, E. N., B. F. Anderson, H. M. Baker, C. L. Day, M. Haridas, G. E. Norris, S. V. Rumball, C. A. Smith, and D. H. Thomas. 1994. Three-dimensional structure of lactoferrin in various functional states. *Adv Exp Med Biol* 357:1-12.

[21] Baker, E. N., H. M. Baker, and R. D. Kidd. 2002. Lactoferrin and transferrin: functional variations on a common structural framework. *Biochem Cell Biol* 80:27-34.

[22] Baker, H. M., and E. N. Baker. 2004. Lactoferrin and iron: structural and dynamic aspects of binding and release. *Biometals* 17:209-16.

[23] Baker, M. A., W. L. Maloy, M. Zasloff, and L. S. Jacob. 1993. Anticancer efficacy of Magainin2 and analogue peptides. *Cancer Res* 53:3052-7.

[24] Barth, H., C. Schafer, M. I. Adah, F. Zhang, R. J. Linhardt, H. Toyoda, A. Kinoshita-Toyoda, T. Toida, T. H. Van Kuppevelt, E. Depla, F. Von Weizsacker, H. E. Blum, and T. F. Baumert. 2003. Cellular binding of hepatitis C virus envelope glycoprotein E2 requires cell surface heparan sulfate. *J Biol Chem* 278:41003-12.

[25] Beaumont, S. L., D. J. Maggs, and H. E. Clarke. 2003. Effects of bovine lactoferrin on in vitro replication of feline herpesvirus. *Vet Ophthalmol* 6:245-50.

[26] Belaid, A., M. Aouni, R. Khelifa, A. Trabelsi, M. Jemmali, and K. Hani. 2002. In vitro antiviral activity of dermaseptins against herpes simplex virus type 1. *J Med Virol* 66:229-34.

[27] Beljaars, L., H. I. Bakker, B. W. van der Strate, C. Smit, A. M. Duijvestijn, D. K. Meijer, and G. Molema. 2002. The antiviral protein human lactoferrin is distributed in the body to cytomegalovirus (CMV) infection-prone cells and tissues. *Pharm Res* 19:54-62.

[28] Beljaars, L., B. W. van der Strate, H. I. Bakker, C. Reker-Smit, A. M. van Loenen-Weemaes, F. C. Wiegmans, M. C. Harmsen, G. Molema, and D. K. Meijer. 2004. Inhibition of cytomegalovirus infection by lactoferrin in vitro and in vivo. *Antiviral Res* 63:197-208.

[29] Bellamy, W., M. Takase, H. Wakabayashi, K. Kawase, and M. Tomita. 1992. Antibacterial spectrum of lactoferricin B, a potent bactericidal peptide derived from the N-terminal region of bovine lactoferrin. *J Appl Bacteriol* 73:472-9.

[30] Bellamy, W., M. Takase, K. Yamauchi, H. Wakabayashi, K. Kawase, and M. Tomita. 1992. Identification of the bactericidal domain of lactoferrin. *Biochim Biophys Acta* 1121:130-6.

[31] Bellamy, W., H. Wakabayashi, M. Takase, K. Kawase, S. Shimamura, and M. Tomita. 1993. Killing of Candida albicans by lactoferricin B, a potent antimicrobial peptide derived from the N-terminal region of bovine lactoferrin. *Med Microbiol Immunol* (Berl) 182:97-105.

[32] Bellamy, W. R., H. Wakabayashi, M. Takase, K. Kawase, S. Shimamura, and M. Tomita. 1993. Role of cell-binding in the antibacterial mechanism of lactoferricin B. *J Appl Bacteriol* 75:478-84.

[33] Benne, C. A., C. A. Kraaijeveld, J. A. van Strijp, E. Brouwer, M. Harmsen, J. Verhoef, L. M. van Golde, and J. F. van Iwaarden. 1995. Interactions of surfactant protein A with influenza A viruses: binding and neutralization. *J Infect Dis* 171:335-41.

[34] Berkhout, B., R. Floris, I. Recio, and S. Visser. 2004. The antiviral activity of the milk protein lactoferrin against the human immunodeficiency virus type 1. *Biometals* 17:291-4.

[35] Berkhout, B., J. L. van Wamel, L. Beljaars, D. K. Meijer, S. Visser, and R. Floris. 2002. Characterization of the anti-HIV effects of native lactoferrin and other milk proteins and protein-derived peptides. *Antiviral Res* 55:341-55.

[36] Berlutti, F., C. Morea, A. Battistoni, S. Sarli, P. Cipriani, F. Superti, M. G. Ammendolia, and P. Valenti. 2005. Iron availability influences aggregation, biofilm, adhesion and invasion of Pseudomonas aeruginosa and Burkholderia cenocepacia. *Int J Immunopathol Pharmacol* 18:661-70.

[37] Bernfield, M., R. Kokenyesi, M. Kato, M. T. Hinkes, J. Spring, R. L. Gallo, and E. J. Lose. 1992. Biology of the syndecans: a family of transmembrane heparan sulfate proteoglycans. *Annu Rev Cell Biol* 8:365-93.

[38] Birgens, H. S., N. E. Hansen, H. Karle, and L. O. Kristensen. 1983. Receptor binding of lactoferrin by human monocytes. *Br J Haematol* 54:383-91.

[39] Blocker, A., P. Gounon, E. Larquet, K. Niebuhr, V. Cabiaux, C. Parsot, and P. Sansonetti. 1999. The tripartite type III secreton of Shigella flexneri inserts IpaB and IpaC into host membranes. *J Cell Biol* 147:683-93.

[40] Boman, H. G. 1995. Peptide antibiotics and their role in innate immunity. *Annu Rev Immunol* 13:61-92.

[41] Boman, H. G., B. Agerberth, and A. Boman. 1993. Mechanisms of action on Escherichia coli of cecropin P1 and PR-39, two antibacterial peptides from pig intestine. *Infect Immun* 61:2978-84.

[42] Bortner, C. A., R. R. Arnold, and R. D. Miller. 1989. Bactericidal effect of lactoferrin on Legionella pneumophila: effect of the physiological state of the organism. *Can J Microbiol* 35:1048-51.

[43] Bousarghin, L., A. Touze, A. L. Combita-Rojas, and P. Coursaget. 2003. Positively charged sequences of human papillomavirus type 16 capsid proteins are sufficient to mediate gene transfer into target cells via the heparan sulfate receptor. *J Gen Virol* 84:157-64.

[44] Bowdish, D. M., D. J. Davidson, and R. E. W. Hancock. 2005. A re-evaluation of the role of host defence peptides in mammalian immunity. *Curr Protein Pept Sci* 6:35-51.

[45] Bowdish, D. M., D. J. Davidson, D. P. Speert, and R. E. W. Hancock. 2004. The human cationic peptide LL-37 induces activation of the extracellular signal-regulated kinase and p38 kinase pathways in primary human monocytes. *J Immunol* 172:3758-65.

[46] Brandenburg, K., G. Jurgens, M. Muller, S. Fukuoka, and M. H. Koch. 2001. Biophysical characterization of lipopolysaccharide and lipid A inactivation by lactoferrin. *Biol Chem* 382:1215-25.

[47] Brantl, V., H. Teschemacher, A. Henschen, and F. Lottspeich. 1979. Novel opioid peptides derived from casein (beta-casomorphins). I. Isolation from bovine casein peptone. *Hoppe Seylers Z Physiol Chem* 360:1211-6.

[48] Brines, R. D., and J. H. Brock. 1983. The effect of trypsin and chymotrypsin on the in vitro antimicrobial and iron-binding properties of lactoferrin in human milk and bovine colostrum. Unusual resistance of human apolactoferrin to proteolytic digestion. *Biochim Biophys Acta* 759:229-35.

[49] Britton, J. R., and O. Koldovsky. 1989. Gastric luminal digestion of lactoferrin and transferrin by preterm infants. *Early Hum Dev* 19:127-35.

[50] Brock, J. 1995. Lactoferrin: a multifunctional immunoregulatory protein? *Immunol Today* 16:417-9.

[51] Brock, J. H. 2002. The physiology of lactoferrin. *Biochem Cell Biol* 80:1-6.

[52] Brogan, T. D., H. C. Ryley, L. Neale, and J. Yassa. 1975. Soluble proteins of bronchopulmonary secretions from patients with cystic fibrosis, asthma, and bronchitis. *Thorax* 30:72-9.

[53] Brogden, K. A. 2005. Antimicrobial peptides: pore formers or metabolic inhibitors in bacteria? *Nat Rev Microbiol* 3:238-50.

[54] Bullen, J. J., H. J. Rogers, and L. Leigh. 1972. Iron-binding proteins in milk and resistance to Escherichia coli infection in infants. *Br Med J* 1:69-75.

[55] Buttner, D., and U. Bonas. 2002. Port of entry--the type III secretion translocon. *Trends Microbiol* 10:186-92.

[56] Camejo, E. H., B. Rosengren, G. Camejo, P. Sartipy, G. Fager, and G. Bondjers. 1995. Interferon gamma binds to extracellular matrix chondroitin-sulfate proteoglycans, thus enhancing its cellular response. *Arterioscler Thromb Vasc Biol* 15:1456-65.

[57] Cappelli, G., S. Paladini, and A. D'Agata. 1999. Tumor markers in the diagnosis of pancreatic cancer. *Tumori* 85:S19-21.

[58] Castle, M., A. Nazarian, S. S. Yi, and P. Tempst. 1999. Lethal effects of apidaecin on Escherichia coli involve sequential molecular interactions with diverse targets. *J Biol Chem* 274:32555-64.

[59] Chan, Y. R., and R. L. Gallo. 1998. PR-39, a syndecan-inducing antimicrobial peptide, binds and affects p130(Cas). *J Biol Chem* 273:28978-85.

[60] Chang, T. L., J. Vargas, Jr., A. DelPortillo, and M. E. Klotman. 2005. Dual role of alpha-defensin-1 in anti-HIV-1 innate immunity. *J Clin Invest* 115:765-73.

[61] Chapple, D. S., R. Hussain, C. L. Joannou, R. E. W. Hancock, E. Odell, R. W. Evans, and G. Siligardi. 2004. Structure and association of human lactoferrin peptides with Escherichia coli lipopolysaccharide. *Antimicrob Agents Chemother* 48:2190-8.

[62] Chapple, D. S., D. J. Mason, C. L. Joannou, E. W. Odell, V. Gant, and R. W. Evans. 1998. Structure-function relationship of antibacterial synthetic peptides homologous to a helical surface region on human lactoferrin against Escherichia coli serotype O111. *Infect Immun* 66:2434-40.

[63] Chen, H. L., Y. W. Lai, C. C. Yen, Y. Y. Lin, C. Y. Lu, S. H. Yang, T. C. Tsai, Y. J. Lin, C. W. Lin, and C. M. Chen. 2004. Production of recombinant porcine lactoferrin exhibiting antibacterial activity in methylotrophic yeast, Pichia pastoris. *J Mol Microbiol Biotechnol* 8:141-9.

[64] Chen, H. L., C. C. Yen, C. Y. Lu, C. H. Yu, and C. M. Chen. 2006. Synthetic porcine lactoferricin with a 20-residue peptide exhibits antimicrobial activity against Escherichia coli, Staphylococcus aureus, and Candida albicans. *J Agric Food Chem* 54:3277-82.

[65] Chen, H. M., W. Wang, D. Smith, and S. C. Chan. 1997. Effects of the anti-bacterial peptide cecropin B and its analogs, cecropins B-1 and B-2, on liposomes, bacteria, and cancer cells. *Biochim Biophys Acta* 1336:171-9.

[66] Chertov, O., D. F. Michiel, L. Xu, J. M. Wang, K. Tani, W. J. Murphy, D. L. Longo, D. D. Taub, and J. J. Oppenheim. 1996. Identification of defensin-1, defensin-2, and CAP37/azurocidin as T-cell chemoattractant proteins released from interleukin-8-stimulated neutrophils. *J Biol Chem* 271:2935-40.

[67] Cheshenko, N., and B. C. Herold. 2002. Glycoprotein B plays a predominant role in mediating herpes simplex virus type 2 attachment and is required for entry and cell-to-cell spread. *J Gen Virol* 83:2247-55.

[68] Cirioni, O., A. Giacometti, F. Barchiesi, and G. Scalise. 2000. Inhibition of growth of Pneumocystis carinii by lactoferrins alone and in combination

with pyrimethamine, clarithromycin and minocycline. *J Antimicrob Chemother* 46:577-82.

[69] Combita, A. L., A. Touze, L. Bousarghin, P. Y. Sizaret, N. Munoz, and P. Coursaget. 2001. Gene transfer using human papillomavirus pseudovirions varies according to virus genotype and requires cell surface heparan sulfate. *FEMS Microbiol Lett* 204:183-8.

[70] Conneely, O. M. 2001. Antiinflammatory activities of lactoferrin. *J Am Coll Nutr* 20:389S-395S; discussion 396S-397S.

[71] Crouch, S. P., K. J. Slater, and J. Fletcher. 1992. Regulation of cytokine release from mononuclear cells by the iron-binding protein lactoferrin. *Blood* 80:235-40.

[72] Cruciani, R. A., J. L. Barker, M. Zasloff, H. C. Chen, and O. Colamonici. 1991. Antibiotic magainins exert cytolytic activity against transformed cell lines through channel formation. *Proc Natl Acad Sci U S A* 88:3792-6.

[73] Daher, K. A., M. E. Selsted, and R. I. Lehrer. 1986. Direct inactivation of viruses by human granulocyte defensins. *J Virol* 60:1068-74.

[74] Dalmastri, C., P. Valenti, P. Visca, P. Vittorioso, and N. Orsi. 1988. Enhanced antimicrobial activity of lactoferrin by binding to the bacterial surface. *Microbiologica* 11:225-30.

[75] Dathe, M., and T. Wieprecht. 1999. Structural features of helical antimicrobial peptides: their potential to modulate activity on model membranes and biological cells. *Biochim Biophys Acta* 1462:71-87.

[76] Davidson, D. J., A. J. Currie, G. S. Reid, D. M. Bowdish, K. L. MacDonald, R. C. Ma, R. E. W. Hancock, and D. P. Speert. 2004. The cationic antimicrobial peptide LL-37 modulates dendritic cell differentiation and dendritic cell-induced T cell polarization. *J Immunol* 172:1146-56.

[77] Davidson, L. A., and B. Lonnerdal. 1986. Isolation and characterization of rhesus monkey milk lactoferrin. *Pediatr Res* 20:197-201.

[78] Davies, J. S., C. Enjalbal, C. Wise, G. Jones, and B. K. Handa. 1994. Further studies on cyclic RGD analogues. *Biochem Soc Trans* 22:1049-52.

[79] De Lucca, A. J., and T. J. Walsh. 1999. Antifungal peptides: novel therapeutic compounds against emerging pathogens. *Antimicrob Agents Chemother* 43:1-11.

[80] Dhaenens, L., F. Szczebara, and M. O. Husson. 1997. Identification, characterization, and immunogenicity of the lactoferrin-binding protein from Helicobacter pylori. *Infect Immun* 65:514-8.

[81] Di Biase, A. M., A. Pietrantoni, A. Tinari, R. Siciliano, P. Valenti, G. Antonini, L. Seganti, and F. Superti. 2003. Heparin-interacting sites of

bovine lactoferrin are involved in anti-adenovirus activity. *J Med Virol* 69:495-502.

[82] DiGabriele, A. D., I. Lax, D. I. Chen, C. M. Svahn, M. Jaye, J. Schlessinger, and W. A. Hendrickson. 1998. Structure of a heparin-linked biologically active dimer of fibroblast growth factor. *Nature* 393:812-7.

[83] Dionysius, D. A., and J. M. Milne. 1997. Antibacterial peptides of bovine lactoferrin: purification and characterization. *J Dairy Sci* 80:667-74.

[84] Drobni, P., N. Mistry, N. McMillan, and M. Evander. 2003. Carboxy-fluorescein diacetate, succinimidyl ester labeled papillomavirus virus-like particles fluoresce after internalization and interact with heparan sulfate for binding and entry. *Virology* 310:163-72.

[85] Drobni, P., J. Naslund, and M. Evander. 2004. Lactoferrin inhibits human papillomavirus binding and uptake in vitro. *Antiviral Res* 64:63-8.

[86] Ehrenstein, G., and H. Lecar. 1977. Electrically gated ionic channels in lipid bilayers. *Q Rev Biophys* 10:1-34.

[87] Ekins, A., A. G. Khan, S. R. Shouldice, and A. B. Schryvers. 2004. Lactoferrin receptors in gram-negative bacteria: insights into the iron acquisition process. *Biometals* 17:235-43.

[88] Elass-Rochard, E., A. Roseanu, D. Legrand, M. Trif, V. Salmon, C. Motas, J. Montreuil, and G. Spik. 1995. Lactoferrin-lipopolysaccharide interaction: involvement of the 28-34 loop region of human lactoferrin in the high-affinity binding to Escherichia coli 055B5 lipopolysaccharide. *Biochem J* 312 (Pt 3):839-45.

[89] Eliassen, L. T., G. Berge, A. Leknessund, M. Wikman, I. Lindin, C. Lokke, F. Ponthan, J. I. Johnsen, B. Sveinbjornsson, P. Kogner, T. Flaegstad, and O. Rekdal. 2006. The antimicrobial peptide, lactoferricin B, is cytotoxic to neuroblastoma cells in vitro and inhibits xenograft growth in vivo. *Int J Cancer* 119:493-500.

[90] Eliassen, L. T., G. Berge, B. Sveinbjornsson, J. S. Svendsen, L. H. Vorland, and O. Rekdal. 2002. Evidence for a direct antitumor mechanism of action of bovine lactoferricin. *Anticancer Res* 22:2703-10.

[91] Ellerby, H. M., W. Arap, L. M. Ellerby, R. Kain, R. Andrusiak, G. D. Rio, S. Krajewski, C. R. Lombardo, R. Rao, E. Ruoslahti, D. E. Bredesen, and R. Pasqualini. 1999. Anti-cancer activity of targeted pro-apoptotic peptides. *Nat Med* 5:1032-8.

[92] Ellison, R. T., 3rd, and T. J. Giehl. 1991. Killing of gram-negative bacteria by lactoferrin and lysozyme. *J Clin Invest* 88:1080-91.

[93] Ellison, R. T., 3rd, T. J. Giehl, and F. M. LaForce. 1988. Damage of the outer membrane of enteric gram-negative bacteria by lactoferrin and transferrin. *Infect Immun* 56:2774-81.

[94] Ellison, R. T., 3rd, F. M. LaForce, T. J. Giehl, D. S. Boose, and B. E. Dunn. 1990. Lactoferrin and transferrin damage of the gram-negative outer membrane is modulated by Ca2+ and Mg2+. *J Gen Microbiol* 136:1437-46.

[95] Elsbach, P. 2003. What is the real role of antimicrobial polypeptides that can mediate several other inflammatory responses? *J Clin Invest* 111:1643-5.

[96] Epand, R. M., and H. J. Vogel. 1999. Diversity of antimicrobial peptides and their mechanisms of action. *Biochim Biophys Acta* 1462:11-28.

[97] Erdei, J., A. Forsgren, and A. S. Naidu. 1994. Lactoferrin binds to porins OmpF and OmpC in Escherichia coli. *Infect Immun* 62:1236-40.

[98] Esteban, M. A., A. Rodriguez, A. Cuesta, and J. Meseguer. 2005. Effects of lactoferrin on non-specific immune responses of gilthead seabream (Sparus auratus L.). *Fish Shellfish Immunol* 18:109-24.

[99] Evander, M., I. H. Frazer, E. Payne, Y. M. Qi, K. Hengst, and N. A. McMillan. 1997. Identification of the alpha6 integrin as a candidate receptor for papillomaviruses. *J Virol* 71:2449-56.

[100] Faber, C., H. P. Stallmann, D. M. Lyaruu, U. Joosten, C. von Eiff, A. van Nieuw Amerongen, and P. I. Wuisman. 2005. Comparable efficacies of the antimicrobial peptide human lactoferrin 1-11 and gentamicin in a chronic methicillin-resistant Staphylococcus aureus osteomyelitis model. *Antimicrob Agents Chemother* 49:2438-44.

[101] Farnaud, S., and R. W. Evans. 2003. Lactoferrin--a multifunctional protein with antimicrobial properties. *Mol Immunol* 40:395-405.

[102] Feldman, M. F., and G. R. Cornelis. 2003. The multitalented type III chaperones: all you can do with 15 kDa. *FEMS Microbiol Lett* 219:151-8.

[103] Feng, X. J., J. H. Wang, A. S. Shan, D. Teng, Y. L. Yang, Y. Yao, G. P. Yang, Y. C. Shao, S. Liu, and F. Zhang. 2006. Fusion expression of bovine lactoferricin in Escherichia coli. *Protein Expr Purif* 47:110-7.

[104] Florisa, R., I. Recio, B. Berkhout, and S. Visser. 2003. Antibacterial and antiviral effects of milk proteins and derivatives thereof. *Curr Pharm Des* 9:1257-75.

[105] Ford, M. J. 2001. Molecular evolution of transferrin: evidence for positive selection in salmonids. *Mol Biol Evol* 18:639-47.

[106] Friedrich, C. L., D. Moyles, T. J. Beveridge, and R. E. W. Hancock. 2000. Antibacterial action of structurally diverse cationic peptides on gram-positive bacteria. *Antimicrob Agents Chemother* 44:2086-92.

[107] Friedrich, C. L., A. Rozek, A. Patrzykat, and R. E. W. Hancock. 2001. Structure and mechanism of action of an indolicidin peptide derivative with improved activity against gram-positive bacteria. *J Biol Chem* 276:24015-22.

[108] Frishman, W. H., B. Burns, B. Atac, N. Alturk, B. Altajar, and K. Lerrick. 1995. Novel antiplatelet therapies for treatment of patients with ischemic heart disease: inhibitors of the platelet glycoprotein IIb/IIIa integrin receptor. *Am Heart J* 130:877-92.

[109] Fromm, J. R., R. E. Hileman, E. E. Caldwell, J. M. Weiler, and R. J. Linhardt. 1995. Differences in the interaction of heparin with arginine and lysine and the importance of these basic amino acids in the binding of heparin to acidic fibroblast growth factor. *Arch Biochem Biophys* 323:279-87.

[110] Fuchs, S. M., and R. T. Raines. 2004. Pathway for polyarginine entry into mammalian cells. *Biochemistry* 43:2438-44.

[111] Fujihara, T., and K. Hayashi. 1995. Lactoferrin inhibits herpes simplex virus type-1 (HSV-1) infection to mouse cornea. *Arch Virol* 140:1469-72.

[112] Fujimura, M., M. Ideguchi, Y. Minami, K. Watanabe, and K. Tadera. 2004. Purification, characterization, and sequencing of novel antimicrobial peptides, Tu-AMP 1 and Tu-AMP 2, from bulbs of tulip (Tulipa gesneriana L.). *Biosci Biotechnol Biochem* 68:571-7.

[113] Furlong, S. J., J. S. Mader, and D. W. Hoskin. 2006. Lactoferricin-induced apoptosis in estrogen-nonresponsive MDA-MB-435 breast cancer cells is enhanced by C6 ceramide or tamoxifen. *Oncol Rep* 15:1385-90.

[114] Futaki, S. 2002. Arginine-rich peptides: potential for intracellular delivery of macromolecules and the mystery of the translocation mechanisms. Int J Pharm 245:1-7.

[115] Futaki, S., I. Nakase, T. Suzuki, Z. Youjun, and Y. Sugiura. 2002. Translocation of branched-chain arginine peptides through cell membranes: flexibility in the spatial disposition of positive charges in membrane-permeable peptides. *Biochemistry* 41:7925-30.

[116] Gahr, M., C. P. Speer, B. Damerau, and G. Sawatzki. 1991. Influence of lactoferrin on the function of human polymorphonuclear leukocytes and monocytes. *J Leukoc Biol* 49:427-33.

[117] Ganz, T. 2005. Defensins and other antimicrobial peptides: a historical perspective and an update. *Comb Chem High Throughput Screen* 8:209-17.

[118] Giansanti, F., M. T. Massucci, M. F. Giardi, F. Nozza, E. Pulsinelli, C. Nicolini, D. Botti, and G. Antonini. 2005. Antiviral activity of ovotransferrin derived peptides. *Biochem Biophys Res Commun* 331:69-73.

[119] Gifford, J. L., H. N. Hunter, and H. J. Vogel. 2005. Lactoferricin: a lactoferrin-derived peptide with antimicrobial, antiviral, antitumor and immunological properties. *Cell Mol Life Sci* 62:2588-98.

[120] Giroglou, T., L. Florin, F. Schafer, R. E. Streeck, and M. Sapp. 2001. Human papillomavirus infection requires cell surface heparan sulfate. *J Virol* 75:1565-70.

[121] Goldman, R. C., and A. Branstrom. 1999. Targeting cell wall synthesis and assembly in microbes: similarities and contrasts between bacteria and fungi. *Curr Pharm Des* 5:473-501.

[122] Gomez, H. F., T. J. Ochoa, L. G. Carlin, and T. G. Cleary. 2003. Human lactoferrin impairs virulence of Shigella flexneri. *J Infect Dis* 187:87-95.

[123] Grossmann, J. G., M. Neu, E. Pantos, F. J. Schwab, R. W. Evans, E. Townes-Andrews, P. F. Lindley, H. Appel, W. G. Thies, and S. S. Hasnain. 1992. X-ray solution scattering reveals conformational changes upon iron uptake in lactoferrin, serum and ovo-transferrins. *J Mol Biol* 225:811-9.

[124] Grover, M., O. Giouzeppos, R. D. Schnagl, and J. T. May. 1997. Effect of human milk prostaglandins and lactoferrin on respiratory syncytial virus and rotavirus. *Acta Paediatr* 86:315-6.

[125] Hallock, K. J., D. K. Lee, and A. Ramamoorthy. 2003. MSI-78, an analogue of the magainin antimicrobial peptides, disrupts lipid bilayer structure via positive curvature strain. *Biophys J* 84:3052-60.

[126] Hammerschmidt, S., G. Bethe, P. H. Remane, and G. S. Chhatwal. 1999. Identification of pneumococcal surface protein A as a lactoferrin-binding protein of Streptococcus pneumoniae. *Infect Immun* 67:1683-7.

[127] Hancock, R. E. W. 2001. Cationic peptides: effectors in innate immunity and novel antimicrobials. *Lancet Infect Dis* 1:156-64.

[128] Hancock, R. E. W., and D. S. Chapple. 1999. Peptide antibiotics. *Antimicrob Agents Chemother* 43:1317-23.

[129] Hancock, R. E. W., and G. Diamond. 2000. The role of cationic antimicrobial peptides in innate host defences. *Trends Microbiol* 8:402-10.

[130] Hancock, R. E. W., and A. Patrzykat. 2002. Clinical development of cationic antimicrobial peptides: from natural to novel antibiotics. *Curr Drug Targets Infect Disord* 2:79-83.

[131] Hancock, R. E. W., and A. Rozek. 2002. Role of membranes in the activities of antimicrobial cationic peptides. *FEMS Microbiol Lett* 206:143-9.

[132] Hara, K., M. Ikeda, S. Saito, S. Matsumoto, K. Numata, N. Kato, K. Tanaka, and H. Sekihara. 2002. Lactoferrin inhibits hepatitis B virus infection in cultured human hepatocytes. *Hepatol Res* 24:228.

[133] Haridas, M., B. F. Anderson, H. M. Baker, G. E. Norris, and E. N. Baker. 1994. X-ray structural analysis of bovine lactoferrin at 2.5 A resolution. *Adv Exp Med Biol* 357:235-8.

[134] Harmsen, M. C., P. J. Swart, M. P. de Bethune, R. Pauwels, E. De Clercq, T. H. The, and D. K. Meijer. 1995. Antiviral effects of plasma and milk proteins: lactoferrin shows potent activity against both human immunodeficiency virus and human cytomegalovirus replication in vitro. *J Infect Dis* 172:380-8.

[135] Hasegawa, K., W. Motsuchi, S. Tanaka, and S. Dosako. 1994. Inhibition with lactoferrin of in vitro infection with human herpes virus. *Jpn J Med Sci Biol* 47:73-85.

[136] Haug, B. E., M. L. Skar, and J. S. Svendsen. 2001. Bulky aromatic amino acids increase the antibacterial activity of 15-residue bovine lactoferricin derivatives. *J Pept Sci* 7:425-32.

[137] Haukland, H. H., H. Ulvatne, K. Sandvik, and L. H. Vorland. 2001. The antimicrobial peptides lactoferricin B and magainin 2 cross over the bacterial cytoplasmic membrane and reside in the cytoplasm. *FEBS Lett* 508:389-93.

[138] Haurum, J. S., S. Thiel, I. M. Jones, P. B. Fischer, S. B. Laursen, and J. C. Jensenius. 1993. Complement activation upon binding of mannan-binding protein to HIV envelope glycoproteins. *Aids* 7:1307-13.

[139] He, J., and P. Furmanski. 1995. Sequence specificity and transcriptional activation in the binding of lactoferrin to DNA. *Nature* 373:721-4.

[140] He, K., S. J. Ludtke, D. L. Worcester, and H. W. Huang. 1996. Neutron scattering in the plane of membranes: structure of alamethicin pores. *Biophys J* 70:2659-66.

[141] Hellberg, S., M. Sjostrom, B. Skagerberg, and S. Wold. 1987. Peptide quantitative structure-activity relationships, a multivariate approach. *J Med Chem* 30:1126-35.

[142] Helmerhorst, E. J., R. F. Troxler, and F. G. Oppenheim. 2001. The human salivary peptide histatin 5 exerts its antifungal activity through the formation of reactive oxygen species. *Proc Natl Acad Sci U S A* 98:14637-42.

[143] Hendrixson, D. R., J. Qiu, S. C. Shewry, D. L. Fink, S. Petty, E. N. Baker, A. G. Plaut, and J. W. St Geme, 3rd. 2003. Human milk lactoferrin is a serine protease that cleaves Haemophilus surface proteins at arginine-rich sites. *Mol Microbiol* 47:607-17.

[144] Henschen, A., F. Lottspeich, V. Brantl, and H. Teschemacher. 1979. Novel opioid peptides derived from casein (beta-casomorphins). II. Structure of

active components from bovine casein peptone. *Hoppe Seylers Z Physiol Chem* 360:1217-24.

[145] Henzler Wildman, K. A., D. K. Lee, and A. Ramamoorthy. 2003. Mechanism of lipid bilayer disruption by the human antimicrobial peptide, LL-37. *Biochemistry* 42:6545-58.

[146] Herold, B. C., S. I. Gerber, B. J. Belval, A. M. Siston, and N. Shulman. 1996. Differences in the susceptibility of herpes simplex virus types 1 and 2 to modified heparin compounds suggest serotype differences in viral entry. *J Virol* 70:3461-9.

[147] Herz, J., and D. K. Strickland. 2001. LRP: a multifunctional scavenger and signaling receptor. *J Clin Invest* 108:779-84.

[148] Hileman, R. E., J. R. Fromm, J. M. Weiler, and R. J. Linhardt. 1998. Glycosaminoglycan-protein interactions: definition of consensus sites in glycosaminoglycan binding proteins. *Bioessays* 20:156-67.

[149] Hoek, K. S., J. M. Milne, P. A. Grieve, D. A. Dionysius, and R. Smith. 1997. Antibacterial activity in bovine lactoferrin-derived peptides. *Antimicrob Agents Chemother* 41:54-9.

[150] Hoogewerf, A. J., G. S. Kuschert, A. E. Proudfoot, F. Borlat, I. Clark-Lewis, C. A. Power, and T. N. Wells. 1997. Glycosaminoglycans mediate cell surface oligomerization of chemokines. *Biochemistry* 36:13570-8.

[151] Hovanessian, A. G., F. Puvion-Dutilleul, S. Nisole, J. Svab, E. Perret, J. S. Deng, and B. Krust. 2000. The cell-surface-expressed nucleolin is associated with the actin cytoskeleton. *Exp Cell Res* 261:312-28.

[152] Hsu, C. H., C. Chen, M. L. Jou, A. Y. Lee, Y. C. Lin, Y. P. Yu, W. T. Huang, and S. H. Wu. 2005. Structural and DNA-binding studies on the bovine antimicrobial peptide, indolicidin: evidence for multiple conformations involved in binding to membranes and DNA. *Nucleic Acids Res* 33:4053-64.

[153] Huang, R. H., Y. Xiang, G. Z. Tu, Y. Zhang, and D. C. Wang. 2004. Solution structure of Eucommia antifungal peptide: a novel structural model distinct with a five-disulfide motif. *Biochemistry* 43:6005-12.

[154] Hung, S. L., S. Srinivasan, H. M. Friedman, R. J. Eisenberg, and G. H. Cohen. 1992. Structural basis of C3b binding by glycoprotein C of herpes simplex virus. *J Virol* 66:4013-27.

[155] Hunter, H. N., A. R. Demcoe, H. Jenssen, T. J. Gutteberg, and H. J. Vogel. 2005. Human lactoferricin is partially folded in aqueous solution and is better stabilized in a membrane mimetic solvent. *Antimicrob Agents Chemother* 49:3387-95.

[156] Hunter, H. N., W. Jing, D. J. Schibli, T. Trinh, I. Y. Park, S. C. Kim, and H. J. Vogel. 2005. The interactions of antimicrobial peptides derived from lysozyme with model membrane systems. *Biochim Biophys Acta* 1668:175-89.

[157] Huth, P. J., D. B. DiRienzo, and G. D. Miller. 2006. Major scientific advances with dairy foods in nutrition and health. *J Dairy Sci* 89:1207-21.

[158] Hwang, P. M., N. Zhou, X. Shan, C. H. Arrowsmith, and H. J. Vogel. 1998. Three-dimensional solution structure of lactoferricin B, an antimicrobial peptide derived from bovine lactoferrin. *Biochemistry* 37:4288-98.

[159] Iida, J., A. M. Meijne, T. R. Oegema, Jr., T. A. Yednock, N. L. Kovach, L. T. Furcht, and J. B. McCarthy. 1998. A role of chondroitin sulfate glycosaminoglycan binding site in alpha4beta1 integrin-mediated melanoma cell adhesion. *J Biol Chem* 273:5955-62.

[160] Ikeda, M., A. Nozaki, K. Sugiyama, T. Tanaka, A. Naganuma, K. Tanaka, H. Sekihara, K. Shimotohno, M. Saito, and N. Kato. 2000. Characterization of antiviral activity of lactoferrin against hepatitis C virus infection in human cultured cells. *Virus Res* 66:51-63.

[161] Ikeda, M., K. Sugiyama, T. Tanaka, K. Tanaka, H. Sekihara, K. Shimotohno, and N. Kato. 1998. Lactoferrin markedly inhibits hepatitis C virus infection in cultured human hepatocytes. *Biochem Biophys Res Commun* 245:549-53.

[162] Iozzo, R. V., and A. D. Murdoch. 1996. Proteoglycans of the extracellular environment: clues from the gene and protein side offer novel perspectives in molecular diversity and function. *Faseb J* 10:598-614.

[163] Ishikado, A., H. Imanaka, M. Kotani, A. Fujita, Y. Mitsuishi, T. Kanemitsu, Y. Tamura, and T. Makino. 2004. Liposomal lactoferrin induced significant increase of the interferon-alpha (IFN-alpha) producibility in healthy volunteers. *Biofactors* 21:69-72.

[164] James, S., B. F. Gibbs, K. Toney, and H. P. Bennett. 1994. Purification of antimicrobial peptides from an extract of the skin of Xenopus laevis using heparin-affinity HPLC: characterization by ion-spray mass spectrometry. *Anal Biochem* 217:84-90.

[165] Jarvis, K. G., J. A. Giron, A. E. Jerse, T. K. McDaniel, M. S. Donnenberg, and J. B. Kaper. 1995. Enteropathogenic Escherichia coli contains a putative type III secretion system necessary for the export of proteins involved in attaching and effacing lesion formation. *Proc Natl Acad Sci U S A* 92:7996-8000.

[166] Javadpour, M. M., M. M. Juban, W. C. Lo, S. M. Bishop, J. B. Alberty, S. M. Cowell, C. L. Becker, and M. L. McLaughlin. 1996. De novo

antimicrobial peptides with low mammalian cell toxicity. *J Med Chem* 39:3107-13.

[167] Jenssen, H. 2005. Anti herpes simplex virus activity of lactoferrin/lactoferricin -- an example of antiviral activity of antimicrobial protein/peptide. *Cell Mol Life Sci* 62:3002-13.

[168] Jenssen, H., J. H. Andersen, D. Mantzilas, and T. J. Gutteberg. 2004. A wide range of medium-sized, highly cationic, alpha-helical peptides show antiviral activity against herpes simplex virus. *Antiviral Res* 64:119-26.

[169] Jenssen, H., J. H. Andersen, L. Uhlin-Hansen, T. J. Gutteberg, and O. Rekdal. 2004. Anti-HSV activity of lactoferricin analogues is only partly related to their affinity for heparan sulfate. *Antiviral Res* 61:101-9.

[170] Jenssen, H., T. J. Gutteberg, and T. Lejon. 2005. Modelling of anti-HSV activity of lactoferricin analogues using amino acid descriptors. *J Pept Sci* 11:97-103.

[171] Jenssen, H., T. J. Gutteberg, and T. Lejon. 2006. Modelling the anti-herpes simplex virus activity of small cationic peptides using amino acid descriptors. *J Pept Res* 66 (suppl. 1):48-56.

[172] Jenssen, H., P. Hamill, and R. E. W. Hancock. 2006. Peptide antimicrobial agents. *Clin Microbiol Rev* 19:491-511.

[173] Ji, Z. S., and R. W. Mahley. 1994. Lactoferrin binding to heparan sulfate proteoglycans and the LDL receptor-related protein. Further evidence supporting the importance of direct binding of remnant lipoproteins to HSPG. *Arterioscler Thromb* 14:2025-31.

[174] Johnstone, S. A., K. Gelmon, L. D. Mayer, R. E. W. Hancock, and M. B. Bally. 2000. In vitro characterization of the anticancer activity of membrane-active cationic peptides. I. Peptide-mediated cytotoxicity and peptide-enhanced cytotoxic activity of doxorubicin against wild-type and p-glycoprotein over-expressing tumor cell lines. *Anticancer Drug Des* 15:151-60.

[175] Joyce, J. G., J. S. Tung, C. T. Przysiecki, J. C. Cook, E. D. Lehman, J. A. Sands, K. U. Jansen, and P. M. Keller. 1999. The L1 major capsid protein of human papillomavirus type 11 recombinant virus-like particles interacts with heparin and cell-surface glycosaminoglycans on human keratinocytes. *J Biol Chem* 274:5810-22.

[176] Kai, K., K. Komine, Y. Komine, T. Kuroishi, T. Kozutsumi, J. Kobayashi, M. Ohta, H. Kitamura, and K. Kumagai. 2002. Lactoferrin stimulates A Staphylococcus aureus killing activity of bovine phagocytes in the mammary gland. *Microbiol Immunol* 46:187-94.

[177] Kalmar, J. R., and R. R. Arnold. 1988. Killing of Actinobacillus actinomycetemcomitans by human lactoferrin. *Infect Immun* 56:2552-7.

[178] Kang, J. H., M. K. Lee, K. L. Kim, and K. S. Hahm. 1996. Structure-biological activity relationships of 11-residue highly basic peptide segment of bovine lactoferrin. *Int J Pept Protein Res* 48:357-63.

[179] Kaniga, K., D. Trollinger, and J. E. Galan. 1995. Identification of two targets of the type III protein secretion system encoded by the inv and spa loci of Salmonella typhimurium that have homology to the Shigella IpaD and IpaA proteins. *J Bacteriol* 177:7078-85.

[180] Kanyshkova, T. G., D. V. Semenov, V. N. Buneva, and G. A. Nevinsky. 1999. Human milk lactoferrin binds two DNA molecules with different affinities. *FEBS Lett* 451:235-7.

[181] Kawakami, H., and B. Lonnerdal. 1991. Isolation and function of a receptor for human lactoferrin in human fetal intestinal brush-border membranes. *Am J Physiol* 261:G841-6.

[182] Khan, J. A., P. Kumar, M. Paramasivam, R. S. Yadav, M. S. Sahani, S. Sharma, A. Srinivasan, and T. P. Singh. 2001. Camel lactoferrin, a transferrin-cum-lactoferrin: crystal structure of camel apolactoferrin at 2.6 A resolution and structural basis of its dual role. *J Mol Biol* 309:751-61.

[183] Kim, H. H., W. S. Lee, J. M. Yang, and S. Shin. 2003. Basic peptide system for efficient delivery of foreign genes. *Biochim Biophys Acta* 1640:129-36.

[184] Kirkpatrick, C. H., I. Green, R. R. Rich, and A. L. Schade. 1971. Inhibition of growth of Candida albicans by iron-unsaturated lactoferrin: relation to host-defense mechanisms in chronic mucocutaneous candidiasis. *J Infect Dis* 124:539-44.

[185] Kjellen, L., and U. Lindahl. 1991. Proteoglycans: structures and interactions. *Annu Rev Biochem* 60:443-75.

[186] Koczulla, R., G. von Degenfeld, C. Kupatt, F. Krotz, S. Zahler, T. Gloe, K. Issbrucker, P. Unterberger, M. Zaiou, C. Lebherz, A. Karl, P. Raake, A. Pfosser, P. Boekstegers, U. Welsch, P. S. Hiemstra, C. Vogelmeier, R. L. Gallo, M. Clauss, and R. Bals. 2003. An angiogenic role for the human peptide antibiotic LL-37/hCAP-18. *J Clin Invest* 111:1665-72.

[187] Kolset, S. O., and J. T. Gallagher. 1990. Proteoglycans in haemopoietic cells. *Biochim Biophys Acta* 1032:191-211.

[188] Konishi, M., M. Iwasa, K. Yamauchi, R. Sugimoto, N. Fujita, Y. Kobayashi, S. Watanabe, S. Teraguchi, Y. Adachi, and M. Kaito. 2006. Lactoferrin inhibits lipid peroxidation in patients with chronic hepatitis C. *Hepatol Res.* 36:27-32.

[189] Koradi, R., M. Billeter, and K. Wuthrich. 1996. MOLMOL: a program for display and analysis of macromolecular structures. *J Mol Graph* 14:51-5, 29-32.

[190] Koshlukova, S. E., M. W. Araujo, D. Baev, and M. Edgerton. 2000. Released ATP is an extracellular cytotoxic mediator in salivary histatin 5-induced killing of Candida albicans. *Infect Immun* 68:6848-56.

[191] Koshlukova, S. E., T. L. Lloyd, M. W. Araujo, and M. Edgerton. 1999. Salivary histatin 5 induces non-lytic release of ATP from Candida albicans leading to cell death. *J Biol Chem* 274:18872-9.

[192] Kroemer, G., B. Dallaporta, and M. Resche-Rigon. 1998. The mitochondrial death/life regulator in apoptosis and necrosis. *Annu Rev Physiol* 60:619-42.

[193] Kuhara, T., K. Yamauchi, Y. Tamura, and H. Okamura. 2006. Oral Administration of Lactoferrin Increases NK Cell Activity in Mice via Increased Production of IL-18 and Type I IFN in the Small Intestine. *J Interferon Cytokine Res* 26:489-99.

[194] Kuipers, M. E., H. G. de Vries, M. C. Eikelboom, D. K. Meijer, and P. J. Swart. 1999. Synergistic fungistatic effects of lactoferrin in combination with antifungal drugs against clinical Candida isolates. *Antimicrob Agents Chemother* 43:2635-41.

[195] Kullberg, B. J., M. G. Netea, A. G. Vonk, and J. W. van der Meer. 1999. Modulation of neutrophil function in host defense against disseminated Candida albicans infection in mice. *FEMS Immunol Med Microbiol* 26:299-307.

[196] Kumar, S., and K. L. Bhatia. 1988. Characterization of buffalo lactotransferrin by polyacrylamide gel electrophoresis in 6 M urea. *J Chromatogr* 434:228-31.

[197] Kustanovich, I., D. E. Shalev, M. Mikhlin, L. Gaidukov, and A. Mor. 2002. Structural requirements for potent versus selective cytotoxicity for antimicrobial dermaseptin S4 derivatives. *J Biol Chem* 277:16941-51.

[198] Kuwata, H., T. T. Yip, K. Yamauchi, S. Teraguchi, H. Hayasawa, M. Tomita, and T. W. Hutchens. 1998. The survival of ingested lactoferrin in the gastrointestinal tract of adult mice. *Biochem J* 334 (Pt 2):321-3.

[199] Kyte, J., and R. F. Doolittle. 1982. A simple method for displaying the hydropathic character of a protein. *J Mol Biol* 157:105-32.

[200] Lau, Y. E., A. Rozek, M. G. Scott, D. L. Goosney, D. J. Davidson, and R. E. W. Hancock. 2005. Interaction and cellular localization of the human host defense peptide LL-37 with lung epithelial cells. *Infect Immun* 73:583-91.

[201] Lee, D. G., Y. Park, I. Jin, K. S. Hahm, H. H. Lee, Y. H. Moon, and E. R. Woo. 2004. Structure-antiviral activity relationships of cecropin A-magainin 2 hybrid peptide and its analogues. *J Pept Sci* 10:298-303.

[202] Legrand, D., K. Vigie, E. A. Said, E. Elass, M. Masson, M. C. Slomianny, M. Carpentier, J. P. Briand, J. Mazurier, and A. G. Hovanessian. 2004. Surface nucleolin participates in both the binding and endocytosis of lactoferrin in target cells. *Eur J Biochem* 271:303-17.

[203] Lehrer, R. I., A. Barton, K. A. Daher, S. S. Harwig, T. Ganz, and M. E. Selsted. 1989. Interaction of human defensins with Escherichia coli. Mechanism of bactericidal activity. *J Clin Invest* 84:553-61.

[204] Leitch, E. C., and M. D. Willcox. 1999. Elucidation of the antistaphylococcal action of lactoferrin and lysozyme. *J Med Microbiol* 48:867-71.

[205] Leitch, E. C., and M. D. Willcox. 1999. Lactoferrin increases the susceptibility of S. epidermidis biofilms to lysozyme and vancomycin. *Curr Eye Res* 19:12-9.

[206] Levay, P. F., and M. Viljoen. 1995. Lactoferrin: a general review. *Haematologica* 80:252-67.

[207] Lewis, L. A., K. Rohde, M. Gipson, B. Behrens, E. Gray, S. I. Toth, B. A. Roe, and D. W. Dyer. 1998. Identification and molecular analysis of lbpBA, which encodes the two-component meningococcal lactoferrin receptor. *Infect Immun* 66:3017-23.

[208] Li, J., J. F. Revol, E. Naranjo, and R. H. Marchessault. 1996. Effect of electrostatic interaction on phase separation behaviour of chitin crystallite suspensions. *Int J Biol Macromol* 18:177-87.

[209] Lim, D. J., Y. M. Chun, H. Y. Lee, S. K. Moon, K. H. Chang, J. D. Li, and A. Andalibi. 2000. Cell biology of tubotympanum in relation to pathogenesis of otitis media - a review. *Vaccine* 19 Suppl 1:S17-25.

[210] Lin, T. Y., C. Chu, and C. H. Chiu. 2002. Lactoferrin inhibits enterovirus 71 infection of human embryonal rhabdomyosarcoma cells in vitro. *J Infect Dis* 186:1161-4.

[211] Lookene, A., R. Savonen, and G. Olivecrona. 1997. Interaction of lipoproteins with heparan sulfate proteoglycans and with lipoprotein lipase. Studies by surface plasmon resonance technique. *Biochemistry* 36:5267-75.

[212] Lopez-Garcia, B., J. F. Marcos, C. Abad, and E. Perez-Paya. 2004. Stabilisation of mixed peptide/lipid complexes in selective antifungal hexapeptides. *Biochim Biophys Acta* 1660:131-7.

[213] Loukas, S., D. Varoucha, C. Zioudrou, R. A. Streaty, and W. A. Klee. 1983. Opioid activities and structures of alpha-casein-derived exorphins. *Biochemistry* 22:4567-73.

[214] Lupetti, A., A. Paulusma-Annema, S. Senesi, M. Campa, J. T. Van Dissel, and P. H. Nibbering. 2002. Internal thiols and reactive oxygen species in candidacidal activity exerted by an N-terminal peptide of human lactoferrin. *Antimicrob Agents Chemother* 46:1634-9.

[215] Lupetti, A., A. Paulusma-Annema, M. M. Welling, S. Senesi, J. T. van Dissel, and P. H. Nibbering. 2000. Candidacidal activities of human lactoferrin peptides derived from the N terminus. *Antimicrob Agents Chemother* 44:3257-63.

[216] Lustig, F., J. Hoebeke, G. Ostergren-Lunden, F. Velge-Roussel, G. Bondjers, U. Olsson, U. Ruetschi, and G. Fager. 1996. Alternative splicing determines the binding of platelet-derived growth factor (PDGF-AA) to glycosaminoglycans. *Biochemistry* 35:12077-85.

[217] Mader, J. S., J. Salsman, D. M. Conrad, and D. W. Hoskin. 2005. Bovine lactoferricin selectively induces apoptosis in human leukemia and carcinoma cell lines. *Mol Cancer Ther* 4:612-24.

[218] Mai, J. C., Z. Mi, S. H. Kim, B. Ng, and P. D. Robbins. 2001. A proapoptotic peptide for the treatment of solid tumors. *Cancer Res* 61:7709-12.

[219] Mandard, N., P. Sodano, H. Labbe, J. M. Bonmatin, P. Bulet, C. Hetru, M. Ptak, and F. Vovelle. 1998. Solution structure of thanatin, a potent bactericidal and fungicidal insect peptide, determined from proton two-dimensional nuclear magnetic resonance data. *Eur J Biochem* 256:404-10.

[220] Mann, D. M., E. Romm, and M. Migliorini. 1994. Delineation of the glycosaminoglycan-binding site in the human inflammatory response protein lactoferrin. *J Biol Chem* 269:23661-7.

[221] Marchetti, M., C. Longhi, M. P. Conte, S. Pisani, P. Valenti, and L. Seganti. 1996. Lactoferrin inhibits herpes simplex virus type 1 adsorption to Vero cells. *Antiviral Res* 29:221-31.

[222] Marchetti, M., S. Pisani, G. Antonini, P. Valenti, L. Seganti, and N. Orsi. 1998. Metal complexes of bovine lactoferrin inhibit in vitro replication of herpes simplex virus type 1 and 2. *Biometals* 11:89-94.

[223] Marchetti, M., F. Superti, M. G. Ammendolia, P. Rossi, P. Valenti, and L. Seganti. 1999. Inhibition of poliovirus type 1 infection by iron-, manganese- and zinc-saturated lactoferrin. *Med Microbiol Immunol* (Berl) 187:199-204.

[224] Marchetti, M., E. Trybala, F. Superti, M. Johansson, and T. Bergstrom. 2004. Inhibition of herpes simplex virus infection by lactoferrin is

dependent on interference with the virus binding to glycosaminoglycans. *Virology* 318:405-13.

[225] Mardberg, K., E. Trybala, F. Tufaro, and T. Bergstrom. 2002. Herpes simplex virus type 1 glycoprotein C is necessary for efficient infection of chondroitin sulfate-expressing gro2C cells. *J Gen Virol* 83:291-300.

[226] Marr, A. K., W. J. Gooderham, and R. E. W. Hancock. 2006. Antibacterial peptides for therapeutic use: obstacles and realistic outlook. Curr Opin Pharmacol.

[227] Marshall, K. 2004. Therapeutic applications of whey protein. *Altern Med Rev* 9:136-56.

[228] Masson, P., J. F. Heremans, and J. Prignot. 1965. Immunohistochemical localization of the iron-binding protein lactoferrin in human bronchial glands. *Experientia* 21:604-5.

[229] Masson, P. L., and J. F. Heremans. 1971. Lactoferrin in milk from different species. *Comp Biochem Physiol* B 39:119-29.

[230] Masson, P. L., J. F. Heremans, and C. Dive. 1966. Studies of the proteins of secretions from two villous tumours of the rectum. *Gastroenterologia* 105:270-82.

[231] Matsuzaki, K., O. Murase, N. Fujii, and K. Miyajima. 1996. An antimicrobial peptide, magainin 2, induced rapid flip-flop of phospholipids coupled with pore formation and peptide translocation. *Biochemistry* 35:11361-8.

[232] Matsuzaki, K., K. Sugishita, N. Ishibe, M. Ueha, S. Nakata, K. Miyajima, and R. M. Epand. 1998. Relationship of membrane curvature to the formation of pores by magainin 2. *Biochemistry* 37:11856-63.

[233] Mazoyer, E., S. Levy-Toledano, F. Rendu, L. Hermant, H. Lu, A. M. Fiat, P. Jolles, and J. Caen. 1990. KRDS, a new peptide derived from human lactotransferrin, inhibits platelet aggregation and release reaction. *Eur J Biochem* 194:43-9.

[234] Mazurier, J., D. Legrand, W. L. Hu, J. Montreuil, and G. Spik. 1989. Expression of human lactotransferrin receptors in phytohemagglutinin-stimulated human peripheral blood lymphocytes. Isolation of the receptors by antiligand-affinity chromatography. *Eur J Biochem* 179:481-7.

[235] McAbee, D. D., and K. Esbensen. 1991. Binding and endocytosis of apo- and holo-lactoferrin by isolated rat hepatocytes. *J Biol Chem* 266:23624-31.

[236] McCann, K. B., A. Lee, J. Wan, H. Roginski, and M. J. Coventry. 2003. The effect of bovine lactoferrin and lactoferricin B on the ability of feline calicivirus (a norovirus surrogate) and poliovirus to infect cell cultures. *J Appl Microbiol* 95:1026-33.

[237] McKeown, S. T., F. T. Lundy, J. Nelson, D. Lockhart, C. R. Irwin, C. G. Cowan, and J. J. Marley. 2006. The cytotoxic effects of human neutrophil peptide-1 (HNP1) and lactoferrin on oral squamous cell carcinoma (OSCC) in vitro. *Oral Oncol.* 42:685-90

[238] McManus, A. M., N. F. Dawson, J. D. Wade, L. E. Carrington, D. J. Winzor, and D. J. Craik. 2000. Three-dimensional structure of RK-1: a novel alpha-defensin peptide. *Biochemistry* 39:15757-64.

[239] McMillan, N. A., E. Payne, I. H. Frazer, and M. Evander. 1999. Expression of the alpha6 integrin confers papillomavirus binding upon receptor-negative B-cells. *Virology* 261:271-9.

[240] Mettenleiter, T. C. 2002. Brief overview on cellular virus receptors. *Virus Res* 82:3-8.

[241] Mikloska, Z., and A. L. Cunningham. 2001. Alpha and gamma interferons inhibit herpes simplex virus type 1 infection and spread in epidermal cells after axonal transmission. *J Virol* 75:11821-6.

[242] Mistry, N., P. Drobni, J. Naslund, V. G. Sunkari, H. Jenssen, and E. M. 2007. The anti-papillomavirus activity of human and bovine lactoferricin. *Antiviral Res* (In press).

[243] Miyagi, T., T. Wada, K. Yamaguchi, and K. Hata. 2004. Sialidase and malignancy: a minireview. *Glycoconj J* 20:189-98.

[244] Moore, S. A., B. F. Anderson, C. R. Groom, M. Haridas, and E. N. Baker. 1997. Three-dimensional structure of diferric bovine lactoferrin at 2.8 A resolution. *J Mol Biol* 274:222-36.

[245] Murphy, M. E., H. Kariwa, T. Mizutani, H. Tanabe, K. Yoshimatsu, J. Arikawa, and I. Takashima. 2001. Characterization of in vitro and in vivo antiviral activity of lactoferrin and ribavirin upon hantavirus. *J Vet Med Sci* 63:637-45.

[246] Murphy, M. E., H. Kariwa, T. Mizutani, K. Yoshimatsu, J. Arikawa, and I. Takashima. 2000. In vitro antiviral activity of lactoferrin and ribavirin upon hantavirus. *Arch Virol* 145:1571-82.

[247] Nakashima, H., M. Masuda, T. Murakami, Y. Koyanagi, A. Matsumoto, N. Fujii, and N. Yamamoto. 1992. Anti-human immunodeficiency virus activity of a novel synthetic peptide, T22 ([Tyr-5,12, Lys-7]polyphemusin II): a possible inhibitor of virus-cell fusion. *Antimicrob Agents Chemother* 36:1249-55.

[248] Nguyen, L. T., D. J. Schibli, and H. J. Vogel. 2005. Structural studies and model membrane interactions of two peptides derived from bovine lactoferricin. *J Pept Sci* 11:379-89.

[249] Nibbering, P. H., E. Ravensbergen, M. M. Welling, L. A. van Berkel, P. H. van Berkel, E. K. Pauwels, and J. H. Nuijens. 2001. Human lactoferrin and peptides derived from its N terminus are highly effective against infections with antibiotic-resistant bacteria. *Infect Immun* 69:1469-76.

[250] Nikaido, H., and M. Vaara. 1985. Molecular basis of bacterial outer membrane permeability. *Microbiol Rev* 49:1-32.

[251] Nikawa, H., H. Fukushima, S. Makihira, T. Hamada, and L. P. Samaranayake. 2004. Fungicidal effect of three new synthetic cationic peptides against Candida albicans. *Oral Dis* 10:221-8.

[252] Nikawa, H., L. P. Samaranayake, and T. Hamada. 1995. Modulation of the anti-Candida activity of apo-lactoferrin by dietary sucrose and tunicamycin in vitro. *Arch Oral Biol* 40:581-4.

[253] Nikawa, H., L. P. Samaranayake, J. Tenovuo, K. M. Pang, and T. Hamada. 1993. The fungicidal effect of human lactoferrin on Candida albicans and Candida krusei. *Arch Oral Biol* 38:1057-63.

[254] Norris, G. E., B. F. Anderson, and E. N. Baker. 1991. Molecular replacement solution of the structure of apolactoferrin, a protein displaying large-scale conformational change. *Acta Crystallogr* B 47 (Pt 6):998-1004.

[255] Ochoa, T. J., and T. G. Clearly. 2004. Lactoferrin disruption of bacterial type III secretion systems. *Biometals* 17:257-60.

[256] Ochoa, T. J., M. Noguera-Obenza, and T. G. Cleary. 2004. Lactoferrin blocks the initial host cell attachment mechanism of Enteropathogenic E. coli (EPEC). *Adv Exp Med Biol* 554:463-6.

[257] Ochoa, T. J., M. Noguera-Obenza, F. Ebel, C. A. Guzman, H. F. Gomez, and T. G. Cleary. 2003. Lactoferrin impairs type III secretory system function in enteropathogenic Escherichia coli. *Infect Immun* 71:5149-55.

[258] Odeh, R., and J. P. Quinn. 2000. Problem pulmonary pathogens: Pseudomonas aeruinosa. *Semin Respir Crit Care Med* 21:331-9.

[259] Odell, E. W., R. Sarra, M. Foxworthy, D. S. Chapple, and R. W. Evans. 1996. Antibacterial activity of peptides homologous to a loop region in human lactoferrin. *FEBS Lett* 382:175-8.

[260] Ohsaki, Y., A. F. Gazdar, H. C. Chen, and B. E. Johnson. 1992. Antitumor activity of magainin analogues against human lung cancer cell lines. *Cancer Res* 52:3534-8.

[261] Okada, S., K. Tanaka, T. Sato, H. Ueno, S. Saito, T. Okusaka, K. Sato, S. Yamamoto, and T. Kakizoe. 2002. Dose-response trial of lactoferrin in patients with chronic hepatitis C. *Jpn J Cancer Res* 93:1063-9.

[262] Olsson, U., G. Camejo, E. Hurt-Camejo, K. Elfsber, O. Wiklund, and G. Bondjers. 1997. Possible functional interactions of apolipoprotein B-100

segments that associate with cell proteoglycans and the ApoB/E receptor. *Arterioscler Thromb Vasc Biol* 17:149-55.

[263] Omata, Y., M. Satake, R. Maeda, A. Saito, K. Shimazaki, K. Yamauchi, Y. Uzuka, S. Tanabe, T. Sarashina, and T. Mikami. 2001. Reduction of the infectivity of Toxoplasma gondii and Eimeria stiedai sporozoites by treatment with bovine lactoferricin. *J Vet Med Sci* 63:187-90.

[264] Oppenheim, F. G., T. Xu, F. M. McMillian, S. M. Levitz, R. D. Diamond, G. D. Offner, and R. F. Troxler. 1988. Histatins, a novel family of histidine-rich proteins in human parotid secretion. Isolation, characterization, primary structure, and fungistatic effects on Candida albicans. *J Biol Chem* 263:7472-7.

[265] Oyane, A., Y. Yokoyama, M. Uchida, and A. Ito. 2006. The formation of an antibacterial agent-apatite composite coating on a polymer surface using a metastable calcium phosphate solution. *Biomaterials* 27:3295-303.

[266] Park, C. B., H. S. Kim, and S. C. Kim. 1998. Mechanism of action of the antimicrobial peptide buforin II: buforin II kills microorganisms by penetrating the cell membrane and inhibiting cellular functions. *Biochem Biophys Res Commun* 244:253-7.

[267] Park, Y., S. H. Jang, D. G. Lee, and K. S. Hahm. 2004. Antinematodal effect of antimicrobial peptide, PMAP-23, isolated from porcine myeloid against Caenorhabditis elegans. *J Pept Sci* 10:304-11.

[268] Parker, K. H., C. P. Winlove, and A. Maroudas. 1988. The theoretical distributions and diffusivities of small ions in chondroitin sulphate and hyaluronate. *Biophys Chem* 32:271-82.

[269] Patrzykat, A., C. L. Friedrich, L. Zhang, V. Mendoza, and R. E. W. Hancock. 2002. Sublethal Concentrations of Pleurocidin-Derived Antimicrobial Peptides Inhibit Macromolecular Synthesis in Escherichia coli. *Antimicrob. Agents Chemother.* 46:605-614.

[270] Patterson, N. A., J. L. Smith, and M. A. Ozbun. 2005. Human papillomavirus type 31b infection of human keratinocytes does not require heparan sulfate. *J Virol* 79:6838-47.

[271] Penco, S., S. Scarfi, M. Giovine, G. Damonte, E. Millo, B. Villaggio, M. Passalacqua, M. Pozzolini, C. Garre, and U. Benatti. 2001. Identification of an import signal for, and the nuclear localization of, human lactoferrin. *Biotechnol Appl Biochem* 34:151-9.

[272] Pettersson, A., T. Prinz, A. Umar, J. van der Biezen, and J. Tommassen. 1998. Molecular characterization of LbpB, the second lactoferrin-binding protein of Neisseria meningitidis. *Mol Microbiol* 27:599-610.

[273] Pettersson, I., M. Kusche, E. Unger, H. Wlad, L. Nylund, U. Lindahl, and L. Kjellen. 1991. Biosynthesis of heparin. Purification of a 110-kDa mouse mastocytoma protein required for both glucosaminyl N-deacetylation and N-sulfation. *J Biol Chem* 266:8044-9.

[274] Pierce, A., D. Colavizza, M. Benaissa, P. Maes, A. Tartar, J. Montreuil, and G. Spik. 1991. Molecular cloning and sequence analysis of bovine lactotransferrin. *Eur J Biochem* 196:177-84.

[275] Pietrantoni, A., M. G. Ammendolia, A. Tinari, R. Siciliano, P. Valenti, and F. Superti. 2006. Bovine lactoferrin peptidic fragments involved in inhibition of Echovirus 6 in vitro infection. *Antiviral Res* 69:98-106.

[276] Pietrantoni, A., A. M. Di Biase, A. Tinari, M. Marchetti, P. Valenti, L. Seganti, and F. Superti. 2003. Bovine lactoferrin inhibits adenovirus infection by interacting with viral structural polypeptides. *Antimicrob Agents Chemother* 47:2688-91.

[277] Platenburg, G. J., E. P. Kootwijk, P. M. Kooiman, S. L. Woloshuk, J. H. Nuijens, P. J. Krimpenfort, F. R. Pieper, H. A. de Boer, and R. Strijker. 1994. Expression of human lactoferrin in milk of transgenic mice. *Transgenic Res* 3:99-108.

[278] Pollock, J. J., L. Denepitiya, B. J. MacKay, and V. J. Iacono. 1984. Fungistatic and fungicidal activity of human parotid salivary histidine-rich polypeptides on Candida albicans. *Infect Immun* 44:702-7.

[279] Portelli, J., A. Gordon, and J. T. May. 1998. Effect of compounds with antibacterial activities in human milk on respiratory syncytial virus and cytomegalovirus in vitro. *J Med Microbiol* 47:1015-8.

[280] Pouny, Y., D. Rapaport, A. Mor, P. Nicolas, and Y. Shai. 1992. Interaction of antimicrobial dermaseptin and its fluorescently labeled analogues with phospholipid membranes. *Biochemistry* 31:12416-23.

[281] Powers, J. P., A. Rozek, and R. E. W. Hancock. 2004. Structure-activity relationships for the beta-hairpin cationic antimicrobial peptide polyphemusin I. *Biochim Biophys Acta* 1698:239-50.

[282] Powers, J. P., A. Tan, A. Ramamoorthy, and R. E. W. Hancock. 2005. Solution structure and interaction of the antimicrobial polyphemusins with lipid membranes. *Biochemistry* 44:15504-13.

[283] Prinz, T., and J. Tommassen. 2000. Association of iron-regulated outer membrane proteins of Neisseria meningitidis with the RmpM (class 4) protein. *FEMS Microbiol Lett* 183:49-53.

[284] Puddu, P., P. Borghi, S. Gessani, P. Valenti, F. Belardelli, and L. Seganti. 1998. Antiviral effect of bovine lactoferrin saturated with metal ions on

early steps of human immunodeficiency virus type 1 infection. *Int J Biochem Cell Biol* 30:1055-62.

[285] Qiu, J., D. R. Hendrixson, E. N. Baker, T. F. Murphy, J. W. St Geme, 3rd, and A. G. Plaut. 1998. Human milk lactoferrin inactivates two putative colonization factors expressed by Haemophilus influenzae. *Proc Natl Acad Sci U S A* 95:12641-6.

[286] Raval, G. N., D. D. Patel, L. J. Parekh, J. B. Patel, M. H. Shah, and P. S. Patel. 2003. Evaluation of serum sialic acid, sialyltransferase and sialoproteins in oral cavity cancer. *Oral Dis* 9:119-28.

[287] Recio, I., C. J. Slangen, and S. Visser. 2000. Method for the production of antibacterial peptides from biological fluids at an ionic membrane. Application to the isolation of nisin and caprine lactoferricin. *Le Lait* 80:187-195.

[288] Retegui, L. A., N. Moguilevsky, C. F. Castracane, and P. L. Masson. 1984. Uptake of lactoferrin by the liver. I. Role of the reticuloendothelial system as indicated by blockade experiments. *Lab Invest* 50:323-8.

[289] Rey, M. W., S. L. Woloshuk, H. A. deBoer, and F. R. Pieper. 1990. Complete nucleotide sequence of human mammary gland lactoferrin. *Nucleic Acids Res* 18:5288.

[290] Rice, P. J., J. L. Kelley, G. Kogan, H. E. Ensley, J. H. Kalbfleisch, I. W. Browder, and D. L. Williams. 2002. Human monocyte scavenger receptors are pattern recognition receptors for (1-->3)-beta-D-glucans. *J Leukoc Biol* 72:140-6.

[291] Risso, A., E. Braidot, M. C. Sordano, A. Vianello, F. Macri, B. Skerlavaj, M. Zanetti, R. Gennaro, and P. Bernardi. 2002. BMAP-28, an antibiotic peptide of innate immunity, induces cell death through opening of the mitochondrial permeability transition pore. *Mol Cell Biol* 22:1926-35.

[292] Robinson, W. E., Jr., B. McDougall, D. Tran, and M. E. Selsted. 1998. Anti-HIV-1 activity of indolicidin, an antimicrobial peptide from neutrophils. *J Leukoc Biol* 63:94-100.

[293] Rochard, E., D. Legrand, M. Lecocq, R. Hamelin, M. Crepin, J. Montreuil, and G. Spik. 1992. Characterization of lactotransferrin receptor in epithelial cell lines from non-malignant human breast, benign mastopathies and breast carcinomas. *Anticancer Res* 12:2047-51.

[294] Rossi, P., F. Giansanti, A. Boffi, M. Ajello, P. Valenti, E. Chiancone, and G. Antonini. 2002. Ca2+ binding to bovine lactoferrin enhances protein stability and influences the release of bacterial lipopolysaccharide. *Biochem Cell Biol* 80:41-8.

[295] Sakamoto, K., Y. Ito, T. Mori, and K. Sugimura. 2006. Interaction of human lactoferrin with cell adhesion molecules through RGD motif elucidated by lactoferrin-binding epitopes. *J Biol Chem* 281:24472-8.

[296] Salmon, V., D. Legrand, M. C. Slomianny, I. el Yazidi, G. Spik, V. Gruber, P. Bournat, B. Olagnier, D. Mison, M. Theisen, and B. Merot. 1998. Production of human lactoferrin in transgenic tobacco plants. *Protein Expr Purif* 13:127-35.

[297] Samuelsen, O., H. H. Haukland, H. Jenssen, M. Kramer, K. Sandvik, H. Ulvatne, and L. H. Vorland. 2005. Induced resistance to the antimicrobial peptide lactoferricin B in Staphylococcus aureus. *FEBS Lett* 579:3421-6.

[298] Samuelsen, O., H. H. Haukland, B. C. Kahl, C. von Eiff, R. A. Proctor, H. Ulvatne, K. Sandvik, and L. H. Vorland. 2005. Staphylococcus aureus small colony variants are resistant to the antimicrobial peptide lactoferricin B. *J Antimicrob Chemother* 56:1126-9.

[299] Schmidtke, M., A. Karger, A. Meerbach, R. Egerer, A. Stelzner, and V. Makarov. 2003. Binding of a N,N'-bisheteryl derivative of dispirotripiperazine to heparan sulfate residues on the cell surface specifically prevents infection of viruses from different families. *Virology* 311:134-43.

[300] Seganti, L., A. M. Di Biase, M. Marchetti, A. Pietrantoni, A. Tinari, and F. Superti. 2004. Antiviral activity of lactoferrin towards naked viruses. *Biometals* 17:295-9.

[301] Selinka, H. C., T. Giroglou, T. Nowak, N. D. Christensen, and M. Sapp. 2003. Further evidence that papillomavirus capsids exist in two distinct conformations. *J Virol* 77:12961-7.

[302] Selinka, H. C., T. Giroglou, and M. Sapp. 2002. Analysis of the infectious entry pathway of human papillomavirus type 33 pseudovirions. *Virology* 299:279-287.

[303] Selsted, M. E. 2004. Theta-defensins: cyclic antimicrobial peptides produced by binary ligation of truncated alpha-defensins. *Curr Protein Pept Sci* 5:365-71.

[304] Sfeir, R. M., M. Dubarry, P. N. Boyaka, M. Rautureau, and D. Tome. 2004. The mode of oral bovine lactoferrin administration influences mucosal and systemic immune responses in mice. *J Nutr* 134:403-9.

[305] Shafti-Keramat, S., A. Handisurya, E. Kriehuber, G. Meneguzzi, K. Slupetzky, and R. Kirnbauer. 2003. Different heparan sulfate proteoglycans serve as cellular receptors for human papillomaviruses. *J Virol* 77:13125-35.

[306] Shakibaei, M., and U. Frevert. 1996. Dual interaction of the malaria circumsporozoite protein with the low density lipoprotein receptor-related protein (LRP) and heparan sulfate proteoglycans. *J Exp Med* 184:1699-711.

[307] Shau, H., A. Kim, and S. H. Golub. 1992. Modulation of natural killer and lymphokine-activated killer cell cytotoxicity by lactoferrin. *J Leukoc Biol* 51:343-9.

[308] Shieh, M. T., D. WuDunn, R. I. Montgomery, J. D. Esko, and P. G. Spear. 1992. Cell surface receptors for herpes simplex virus are heparan sulfate proteoglycans. *J Cell Biol* 116:1273-81.

[309] Shimazaki, K., K. Oota, K. Nitta, and Y. Ke. 1994. Comparative study of the iron-binding strengths of equine, bovine and human lactoferrins. *J Dairy Res* 61:563-6.

[310] Shimazaki, K., T. Tazume, K. Uji, M. Tanaka, H. Kumura, K. Mikawa, and T. Shimo-Oka. 1998. Properties of a heparin-binding peptide derived from bovine lactoferrin. *J Dairy Sci* 81:2841-9.

[311] Shin, K., H. Wakabayashi, K. Yamauchi, S. Teraguchi, Y. Tamura, M. Kurokawa, and K. Shiraki. 2005. Effects of orally administered bovine lactoferrin and lactoperoxidase on influenza virus infection in mice. *J Med Microbiol* 54:717-23.

[312] Shin, K., K. Yamauchi, S. Teraguchi, H. Hayasawa, M. Tomita, Y. Otsuka, and S. Yamazaki. 1998. Antibacterial activity of bovine lactoferrin and its peptides against enterohaemorrhagic Escherichia coli O157:H7. *Lett Appl Microbiol* 26:407-11.

[313] Shukla, D., J. Liu, P. Blaiklock, N. W. Shworak, X. Bai, J. D. Esko, G. H. Cohen, R. J. Eisenberg, R. D. Rosenberg, and P. G. Spear. 1999. A novel role for 3-O-sulfated heparan sulfate in herpes simplex virus 1 entry. *Cell* 99:13-22.

[314] Siciliano, R., B. Rega, M. Marchetti, L. Seganti, G. Antonini, and P. Valenti. 1999. Bovine lactoferrin peptidic fragments involved in inhibition of herpes simplex virus type 1 infection. *Biochem Biophys Res Commun* 264:19-23.

[315] Singh, P. K., M. R. Parsek, E. P. Greenberg, and M. J. Welsh. 2002. A component of innate immunity prevents bacterial biofilm development. *Nature* 417:552-5.

[316] Singh, P. K., B. F. Tack, P. B. McCray, Jr., and M. J. Welsh. 2000. Synergistic and additive killing by antimicrobial factors found in human airway surface liquid. *Am J Physiol Lung Cell Mol Physiol* 279:L799-805.

[317] Sinha, S., N. Cheshenko, R. I. Lehrer, and B. C. Herold. 2003. NP-1, a rabbit alpha-defensin, prevents the entry and intercellular spread of herpes simplex virus type 2. *Antimicrob Agents Chemother* 47:494-500.

[318] Sinnis, P., T. E. Willnow, M. R. Briones, J. Herz, and V. Nussenzweig. 1996. Remnant lipoproteins inhibit malaria sporozoite invasion of hepatocytes. *J Exp Med* 184:945-54.

[319] Sitaram, N., and R. Nagaraj. 1999. Interaction of antimicrobial peptides with biological and model membranes: structural and charge requirements for activity. *Biochim Biophys Acta* 1462:29-54.

[320] Son, K. N., J. Park, C. K. Chung, D. K. Chung, D. Y. Yu, K. K. Lee, and J. Kim. 2002. Human lactoferrin activates transcription of IL-1beta gene in mammalian cells. *Biochem Biophys Res Commun* 290:236-41.

[321] Song, B. H., G. C. Lee, M. S. Moon, Y. H. Cho, and C. H. Lee. 2001. Human cytomegalovirus binding to heparan sulfate proteoglycans on the cell surface and/or entry stimulates the expression of human leukocyte antigen class I. *J Gen Virol* 82:2405-13.

[322] Song, Y. M., Y. Park, S. S. Lim, S. T. Yang, E. R. Woo, I. S. Park, J. S. Lee, J. I. Kim, K. S. Hahm, Y. Kim, and S. Y. Shin. 2005. Cell selectivity and mechanism of action of antimicrobial model peptides containing peptoid residues. *Biochemistry* 44:12094-106.

[323] Soukka, T., J. Tenovuo, and M. Lenander-Lumikari. 1992. Fungicidal effect of human lactoferrin against Candida albicans. *FEMS Microbiol Lett* 69:223-8.

[324] Spaar, A., C. Munster, and T. Salditt. 2004. Conformation of peptides in lipid membranes studied by x-ray grazing incidence scattering. *Biophys J* 87:396-407.

[325] Spear, P. G. 2004. Herpes simplex virus: receptors and ligands for cell entry. *Cell Microbiol* 6:401-10.

[326] Spillmann, D. 2001. Heparan sulfate: anchor for viral intruders? *Biochimie* 83:811-7.

[327] Stenlund, P., M. J. Lindberg, and L. A. Tibell. 2002. Structural requirements for high-affinity heparin binding: alanine scanning analysis of charged residues in the C-terminal domain of human extracellular superoxide dismutase. *Biochemistry* 41:3168-75.

[328] Strom, M. B., B. E. Haug, O. Rekdal, M. L. Skar, W. Stensen, and J. S. Svendsen. 2002. Important structural features of 15-residue lactoferricin derivatives and methods for improvement of antimicrobial activity. *Biochem Cell Biol* 80:65-74.

[329] Strom, M. B., O. Rekdal, W. Stensen, and J. S. Svendsen. 2001. Increased antibacterial activity of 15-residue murine lactoferricin derivatives. *J Pept Res* 57:127-39.

[330] Strom, M. B., O. Rekdal, and J. S. Svendsen. 2000. Antibacterial activity of 15-residue lactoferricin derivatives. *J Pept Res* 56:265-74.

[331] Strom, M. B., O. Rekdal, and J. S. Svendsen. 2002. The effects of charge and lipophilicity on the antibacterial activity of undecapeptides derived from bovine lactoferricin. *J Pept Sci* 8:36-43.

[332] Subbalakshmi, C., and N. Sitaram. 1998. Mechanism of antimicrobial action of indolicidin. *FEMS Microbiol Lett* 160:91-6.

[333] Superti, F., M. G. Ammendolia, P. Valenti, and L. Seganti. 1997. Antirotaviral activity of milk proteins: lactoferrin prevents rotavirus infection in the enterocyte-like cell line HT-29. *Med Microbiol Immunol* (Berl) 186:83-91.

[334] Superti, F., R. Siciliano, B. Rega, F. Giansanti, P. Valenti, and G. Antonini. 2001. Involvement of bovine lactoferrin metal saturation, sialic acid and protein fragments in the inhibition of rotavirus infection. *Biochim Biophys Acta* 1528:107-15.

[335] Suzuki, T., S. Futaki, M. Niwa, S. Tanaka, K. Ueda, and Y. Sugiura. 2002. Possible existence of common internalization mechanisms among arginine-rich peptides. *J Biol Chem* 277:2437-43.

[336] Suzuki, Y. A., K. Shin, and B. Lonnerdal. 2001. Molecular cloning and functional expression of a human intestinal lactoferrin receptor. *Biochemistry* 40:15771-9.

[337] Swart, P. J., M. E. Kuipers, C. Smit, R. Pauwels, M. P. deBethune, E. de Clercq, D. K. Meijer, and J. G. Huisman. 1996. Antiviral effects of milk proteins: acylation results in polyanionic compounds with potent activity against human immunodeficiency virus types 1 and 2 in vitro. *AIDS Res Hum Retroviruses* 12:769-75.

[338] Tachezy, J., J. Kulda, I. Bahnikova, P. Suchan, J. Razga, and J. Schrevel. 1996. Tritrichomonas foetus: iron acquisition from lactoferrin and transferrin. *Exp Parasitol* 83:216-28.

[339] Takakura, N., H. Wakabayashi, H. Ishibashi, K. Yamauchi, S. Teraguchi, Y. Tamura, H. Yamaguchi, and S. Abe. 2004. Effect of orally administered bovine lactoferrin on the immune response in the oral candidiasis murine model. *J Med Microbiol* 53:495-500.

[340] Takase, K., K. Hagiwara, H. Onodera, Y. Nishizawa, M. Ugaki, T. Omura, S. Numata, K. Akutsu, H. Kumura, and K. Shimazaki. 2005. Constitutive

expression of human lactoferrin and its N-lobe in rice plants to confer disease resistance. *Biochem Cell Biol* 83:239-49.

[341] Takeshima, K., A. Chikushi, K. K. Lee, S. Yonehara, and K. Matsuzaki. 2003. Translocation of analogues of the antimicrobial peptides magainin and buforin across human cell membranes. *J Biol Chem* 278:1310-5.

[342] Tamamura, H., T. Murakami, M. Masuda, A. Otaka, W. Takada, T. Ibuka, H. Nakashima, M. Waki, A. Matsumoto, N. Yamamoto, and et al. 1994. Structure-activity relationships of an anti-HIV peptide, T22. *Biochem Biophys Res Commun* 205:1729-35.

[343] Tamamura, H., A. Otaka, T. Murakami, T. Ishihara, T. Ibuka, M. Waki, A. Matsumoto, N. Yamamoto, and N. Fujii. 1996. Interaction of an anti-HIV peptide, T22, with gp120 and CD4. *Biochem Biophys Res Commun* 219:555-9.

[344] Tanaka, K., M. Ikeda, A. Nozaki, N. Kato, H. Tsuda, S. Saito, and H. Sekihara. 1999. Lactoferrin inhibits hepatitis C virus viremia in patients with chronic hepatitis C: a pilot study. *Jpn J Cancer Res* 90:367-71.

[345] Tanaka, T., S. Nakatani, X. Xuan, H. Kumura, I. Igarashi, and K. Shimazaki. 2003. Antiviral activity of lactoferrin against canine herpesvirus. *Antiviral Res* 60:193-9.

[346] Tanaka, T., Y. Omata, A. Saito, K. Shimazaki, K. Yamauchi, M. Takase, K. Kawase, K. Igarashi, and N. Suzuki. 1995. Toxoplasma gondii: parasiticidal effects of bovine lactoferricin against parasites. *Exp Parasitol* 81:614-7.

[347] Tani, F., K. Iio, H. Chiba, and M. Yoshikawa. 1990. Isolation and characterization of opioid antagonist peptides derived from human lactoferrin. *Agric Biol Chem* 54:1803-10.

[348] Territo, M. C., T. Ganz, M. E. Selsted, and R. Lehrer. 1989. Monocyte-chemotactic activity of defensins from human neutrophils. *J Clin Invest* 84:2017-20.

[349] Tinari, A., A. Pietrantoni, M. G. Ammendolia, P. Valenti, and F. Superti. 2005. Inhibitory activity of bovine lactoferrin against echovirus induced programmed cell death in vitro. *Int J Antimicrob Agents* 25:433-8.

[350] Toka, F. N., C. D. Pack, and B. T. Rouse. 2004. Molecular adjuvants for mucosal immunity. *Immunol Rev* 199:100-12.

[351] Tomita, M., W. Bellamy, M. Takase, K. Yamauchi, H. Wakabayashi, and K. Kawase. 1991. Potent antibacterial peptides generated by pepsin digestion of bovine lactoferrin. *J Dairy Sci* 74:4137-42.

[352] Tomita, M., M. Takase, W. Bellamy, and S. Shimamura. 1994. A review: the active peptide of lactoferrin. *Acta Paediatr Jpn* 36:585-91.

[353] Tomita, M., M. Takase, H. Wakabayashi, and W. Bellamy. 1994. Antimicrobial peptides of lactoferrin. *Adv Exp Med Biol* 357:209-18.

[354] Tomita, M., H. Wakabayashi, K. Yamauchi, S. Teraguchi, and H. Hayasawa. 2002. Bovine lactoferrin and lactoferricin derived from milk: production and applications. *Biochem Cell Biol* 80:109-12.

[355] Trybala, E., T. Bergstrom, B. Svennerholm, S. Jeansson, J. C. Glorioso, and S. Olofsson. 1994. Localization of a functional site on herpes simplex virus type 1 glycoprotein C involved in binding to cell surface heparan sulphate. *J Gen Virol* 75 (Pt 4):743-52.

[356] Trybala, E., J. A. Liljeqvist, B. Svennerholm, and T. Bergstrom. 2000. Herpes simplex virus types 1 and 2 differ in their interaction with heparan sulfate. *J Virol* 74:9106-14.

[357] Trybala, E., S. Olofsson, K. Mardberg, B. Svennerholm, K. Umemoto, J. C. Glorioso, and T. Bergstrom. 2004. Structural and functional features of the polycationic peptide required for inhibition of herpes simplex virus invasion of cells. *Antiviral Res* 62:125-34.

[358] Trybala, E., A. Roth, M. Johansson, J. A. Liljeqvist, E. Rekabdar, O. Larm, and T. Bergstrom. 2002. Glycosaminoglycan-binding ability is a feature of wild-type strains of herpes simplex virus type 1. *Virology* 302:413-9.

[359] Tryon, V. V., and J. B. Baseman. 1987. The acquisition of human lactoferrin by Mycoplasma pneumoniae. *Microb Pathog* 3:437-43.

[360] Tsuda, H., K. Sekine, K. Fujita, and M. Ligo. 2002. Cancer prevention by bovine lactoferrin and underlying mechanisms--a review of experimental and clinical studies. *Biochem Cell Biol* 80:131-6.

[361] Turchany, J. M., S. B. Aley, and F. D. Gillin. 1995. Giardicidal activity of lactoferrin and N-terminal peptides. *Infect Immun* 63:4550-2.

[362] Ueta, E., T. Tanida, and T. Osaki. 2001. A novel bovine lactoferrin peptide, FKCRRWQWRM, suppresses Candida cell growth and activates neutrophils. *J Pept Res* 57:240-9.

[363] Ulvatne, H., O. Samuelsen, H. H. Haukland, M. Kramer, and L. H. Vorland. 2004. Lactoferricin B inhibits bacterial macromolecular synthesis in Escherichia coli and Bacillus subtilis. *FEMS Microbiol Lett* 237:377-84.

[364] Utsugi, T., A. J. Schroit, J. Connor, C. D. Bucana, and I. J. Fidler. 1991. Elevated expression of phosphatidylserine in the outer membrane leaflet of human tumor cells and recognition by activated human blood monocytes. *Cancer Res* 51:3062-6.

[365] Valenti, P., P. Visca, G. Antonini, and N. Orsi. 1985. Antifungal activity of ovotransferrin towards genus Candida. *Mycopathologia* 89:169-75.

[366] van Berkel, P. H., M. E. Geerts, H. A. van Veen, M. Mericskay, H. A. de Boer, and J. H. Nuijens. 1997. N-terminal stretch Arg2, Arg3, Arg4 and Arg5 of human lactoferrin is essential for binding to heparin, bacterial lipopolysaccharide, human lysozyme and DNA. *Biochem J* 328 (Pt 1):145-51.

[367] van Berkel, P. H., M. M. Welling, M. Geerts, H. A. van Veen, B. Ravensbergen, M. Salaheddine, E. K. Pauwels, F. Pieper, J. H. Nuijens, and P. H. Nibbering. 2002. Large scale production of recombinant human lactoferrin in the milk of transgenic cows. *Nat Biotechnol* 20:484-7.

[368] van der Kraan, M. I., J. Groenink, K. Nazmi, E. C. Veerman, J. G. Bolscher, and A. V. Nieuw Amerongen. 2004. Lactoferrampin: a novel antimicrobial peptide in the N1-domain of bovine lactoferrin. *Peptides* 25:177-83.

[369] van der Kraan, M. I., K. Nazmi, A. Teeken, J. Groenink, W. van 't Hof, E. C. Veerman, J. G. Bolscher, and A. V. Nieuw Amerongen. 2005. Lactoferrampin, an antimicrobial peptide of bovine lactoferrin, exerts its candidacidal activity by a cluster of positively charged residues at the C-terminus in combination with a helix-facilitating N-terminal part. *Biol Chem* 386:137-42.

[370] van der Kraan, M. I., J. van Marle, K. Nazmi, J. Groenink, W. van 't Hof, E. C. Veerman, J. G. Bolscher, and A. V. Nieuw Amerongen. 2005. Ultrastructural effects of antimicrobial peptides from bovine lactoferrin on the membranes of Candida albicans and Escherichia coli. *Peptides* 26:1537-42.

[371] van der Strate, B. W., L. Beljaars, G. Molema, M. C. Harmsen, and D. K. Meijer. 2001. Antiviral activities of lactoferrin. *Antiviral Res* 52:225-39.

[372] Veerman, E. C., K. Nazmi, W. Van't Hof, J. G. Bolscher, A. L. Den Hertog, and A. V. Nieuw Amerongen. 2004. Reactive oxygen species play no role in the candidacidal activity of the salivary antimicrobial peptide histatin 5. *Biochem J* 381:447-52.

[373] Viani, R. M., T. J. Gutteberg, J. L. Lathey, and S. A. Spector. 1999. Lactoferrin inhibits HIV-1 replication in vitro and exhibits synergy when combined with zidovudine. *Aids* 13:1273-4.

[374] Viejo-Diaz, M., M. T. Andres, and J. F. Fierro. 2005. Different anti-Candida activities of two human lactoferrin-derived peptides, Lfpep and kaliocin-1. *Antimicrob Agents Chemother* 49:2583-8.

[375] Viejo-Diaz, M., M. T. Andres, and J. F. Fierro. 2004. Modulation of in vitro fungicidal activity of human lactoferrin against Candida albicans by extracellular cation concentration and target cell metabolic activity. *Antimicrob Agents Chemother* 48:1242-8.

[376] Vives, E., P. Brodin, and B. Lebleu. 1997. A truncated HIV-1 Tat protein basic domain rapidly translocates through the plasma membrane and accumulates in the cell nucleus. *J Biol Chem* 272:16010-7.

[377] Vives, R. R., A. Imberty, Q. J. Sattentau, and H. Lortat-Jacob. 2005. Heparan sulfate targets the HIV-1 envelope glycoprotein gp120 coreceptor binding site. *J Biol Chem* 280:21353-7.

[378] Vogel, H. J., D. J. Schibli, W. Jing, E. M. Lohmeier-Vogel, R. F. Epand, and R. M. Epand. 2002. Towards a structure-function analysis of bovine lactoferricin and related tryptophan- and arginine-containing peptides. *Biochem Cell Biol* 80:49-63.

[379] Vogel, L., F. Geluk, H. Jansen, J. Dankert, and L. van Alphen. 1997. Human lactoferrin receptor activity in non-encapsulated Haemophilus influenzae. *FEMS Microbiol Lett* 156:165-70.

[380] Vorland, L. H. 1999. Lactoferrin: a multifunctional glycoprotein. *Apmis* 107:971-81.

[381] Vorland, L. H., H. Ulvatne, J. Andersen, H. Haukland, O. Rekdal, J. S. Svendsen, and T. J. Gutteberg. 1998. Lactoferricin of bovine origin is more active than lactoferricins of human, murine and caprine origin. *Scand J Infect Dis* 30:513-7.

[382] Vorland, L. H., H. Ulvatne, O. Rekdal, and J. S. Svendsen. 1999. Initial binding sites of antimicrobial peptides in Staphylococcus aureus and Escherichia coli. *Scand J Infect Dis* 31:467-73.

[383] Waarts, B. L., O. J. Aneke, J. M. Smit, K. Kimata, R. Bittman, D. K. Meijer, and J. Wilschut. 2005. Antiviral activity of human lactoferrin: inhibition of alphavirus interaction with heparan sulfate. *Virology* 333:284-92.

[384] Wachinger, M., A. Kleinschmidt, D. Winder, N. von Pechmann, A. Ludvigsen, M. Neumann, R. Holle, B. Salmons, V. Erfle, and R. Brack-Werner. 1998. Antimicrobial peptides melittin and cecropin inhibit replication of human immunodeficiency virus 1 by suppressing viral gene expression. *J Gen Virol* 79 (Pt 4):731-40.

[385] Wakabayashi, H., S. Abe, T. Okutomi, S. Tansho, K. Kawase, and H. Yamaguchi. 1996. Cooperative anti-Candida effects of lactoferrin or its peptides in combination with azole antifungal agents. *Microbiol Immunol* 40:821-5.

[386] Wakabayashi, H., M. Kurokawa, K. Shin, S. Teraguchi, Y. Tamura, and K. Shiraki. 2004. Oral lactoferrin prevents body weight loss and increases cytokine responses during herpes simplex virus type 1 infection of mice. *Biosci Biotechnol Biochem* 68:537-44.

[387] Wakabayashi, H., M. Takase, and M. Tomita. 2003. Lactoferricin derived from milk protein lactoferrin. *Curr Pharm Des* 9:1277-87.

[388] Wang, Z., and G. Wang. 2004. APD: the Antimicrobial Peptide Database. *Nucleic Acids Res* 32:D590-2.

[389] Ward, P. P., X. Zhou, and O. M. Conneely. 1996. Cooperative interactions between the amino- and carboxyl-terminal lobes contribute to the unique iron-binding stability of lactoferrin. *J Biol Chem* 271:12790-4.

[390] Weinberg, E. D. 2001. Human lactoferrin: a novel therapeutic with broad spectrum potential. *J Pharm Pharmacol* 53:1303-10.

[391] Weinberg, E. D. 2004. Suppression of bacterial biofilm formation by iron limitation. *Med Hypotheses* 63:863-5.

[392] Weinberg, G. A. 1994. Iron chelators as therapeutic agents against Pneumocystis carinii. *Antimicrob Agents Chemother* 38:997-1003.

[393] Weng, T. Y., L. C. Chen, H. W. Shyu, S. H. Chen, J. R. Wang, C. K. Yu, H. Y. Lei, and T. M. Yeh. 2005. Lactoferrin inhibits enterovirus 71 infection by binding to VP1 protein and host cells. *Antiviral Res* 67:31-7.

[394] Williamson, P., and R. A. Schlegel. 1994. Back and forth: the regulation and function of transbilayer phospholipid movement in eukaryotic cells. *Mol Membr Biol* 11:199-216.

[395] Wolf, J. S., D. Li, R. J. Taylor, and B. W. O'Malley, Jr. 2003. Lactoferrin inhibits growth of malignant tumors of the head and neck. *ORL J Otorhinolaryngol Relat Spec* 65:245-9.

[396] Wu, H. F., D. M. Monroe, and F. C. Church. 1995. Characterization of the glycosaminoglycan-binding region of lactoferrin. *Arch Biochem Biophys* 317:85-92.

[397] Wu, M., E. Maier, R. Benz, and R. E. W. Hancock. 1999. Mechanism of interaction of different classes of cationic antimicrobial peptides with planar bilayers and with the cytoplasmic membrane of Escherichia coli. *Biochemistry* 38:7235-42.

[398] WuDunn, D., and P. G. Spear. 1989. Initial interaction of herpes simplex virus with cells is binding to heparan sulfate. *J Virol* 63:52-8.

[399] Xia, G., J. Chen, V. Tiwari, W. Ju, J. P. Li, A. Malmstrom, D. Shukla, and J. Liu. 2002. Heparan sulfate 3-O-sulfotransferase isoform 5 generates both an antithrombin-binding site and an entry receptor for herpes simplex virus, type 1. *J Biol Chem* 277:37912-9.

[400] Xu, Y. Y., Y. H. Samaranayake, L. P. Samaranayake, and H. Nikawa. 1999. In vitro susceptibility of Candida species to lactoferrin. *Med Mycol* 37:35-41.

[401] Yalcin, A. S. 2006. Emerging therapeutic potential of whey proteins and peptides. *Curr Pharm Des* 12:1637-43.

[402] Yamaguchi, H., S. Abe, and N. Takakura. 2004. Potential usefulness of bovine lactoferrin for adjunctive immunotherapy for mucosal Candida infections. *Biometals* 17:245-8.

[403] Yamaguchi, S., D. Huster, A. Waring, R. I. Lehrer, W. Kearney, B. F. Tack, and M. Hong. 2001. Orientation and dynamics of an antimicrobial peptide in the lipid bilayer by solid-state NMR spectroscopy. *Biophys J* 81:2203-14.

[404] Yamauchi, K., M. Tomita, T. J. Giehl, and R. T. Ellison, 3rd. 1993. Antibacterial activity of lactoferrin and a pepsin-derived lactoferrin peptide fragment. *Infect Immun* 61:719-28.

[405] Yang, D., A. Biragyn, L. W. Kwak, and J. J. Oppenheim. 2002. Mammalian defensins in immunity: more than just microbicidal. *Trends Immunol* 23:291-6.

[406] Yang, L., T. A. Harroun, T. M. Weiss, L. Ding, and H. W. Huang. 2001. Barrel-Stave Model or Toroidal Model? A Case Study on Melittin Pores. *Biophys. J.* 81:1475-1485.

[407] Yang, N., T. Lejon, and O. Rekdal. 2003. Antitumour activity and specificity as a function of substitutions in the lipophilic sector of helical lactoferrin-derived peptide. *J Pept Sci* 9:300-11.

[408] Yang, N., W. Stensen, J. S. Svendsen, and O. Rekdal. 2002. Enhanced antitumor activity and selectivity of lactoferrin-derived peptides. *J Pept Res* 60:187-97.

[409] Yang, N., M. B. Strom, S. M. Mekonnen, J. S. Svendsen, and O. Rekdal. 2004. The effects of shortening lactoferrin derived peptides against tumour cells, bacteria and normal human cells. *J Pept Sci* 10:37-46.

[410] Yasin, B., M. Pang, J. S. Turner, Y. Cho, N. N. Dinh, A. J. Waring, R. I. Lehrer, and E. A. Wagar. 2000. Evaluation of the inactivation of infectious Herpes simplex virus by host-defense peptides. *Eur J Clin Microbiol Infect Dis* 19:187-94.

[411] Yasin, B., W. Wang, M. Pang, N. Cheshenko, T. Hong, A. J. Waring, B. C. Herold, E. A. Wagar, and R. I. Lehrer. 2004. Theta defensins protect cells from infection by herpes simplex virus by inhibiting viral adhesion and entry. *J Virol* 78:5147-56.

[412] Yi, M., S. Kaneko, D. Y. Yu, and S. Murakami. 1997. Hepatitis C virus envelope proteins bind lactoferrin. *J Virol* 71:5997-6002.

[413] Yoo, Y. C., R. Watanabe, Y. Koike, M. Mitobe, K. Shimazaki, S. Watanabe, and I. Azuma. 1997. Apoptosis in human leukemic cells induced

by lactoferricin, a bovine milk protein-derived peptide: involvement of reactive oxygen species. *Biochem Biophys Res Commun* 237:624-8.

[414] Yoo, Y. C., S. Watanabe, R. Watanabe, K. Hata, K. Shimazaki, and I. Azuma. 1998. Bovine lactoferrin and Lactoferricin inhibit tumor metastasis in mice. *Adv Exp Med Biol* 443:285-91.

[415] Yoo, Y. C., S. Watanabe, R. Watanabe, K. Hata, K. Shimazaki, and I. Azuma. 1997. Bovine lactoferrin and lactoferricin, a peptide derived from bovine lactoferrin, inhibit tumor metastasis in mice. *Jpn J Cancer Res* 88:184-90.

[416] Yoon, C. S., K. D. Kim, S. N. Park, and S. W. Cheong. 2001. alpha(6) Integrin is the main receptor of human papillomavirus type 16 VLP. *Biochem Biophys Res Commun* 283:668-73.

[417] Zasloff, M. 1987. Magainins, a class of antimicrobial peptides from Xenopus skin: isolation, characterization of two active forms, and partial cDNA sequence of a precursor. *Proc Natl Acad Sci U S A* 84:5449-53.

[418] Zautner, A. E., U. Korner, A. Henke, C. Badorff, and M. Schmidtke. 2003. Heparan sulfates and coxsackievirus-adenovirus receptor: each one mediates coxsackievirus B3 PD infection. *J Virol* 77:10071-7.

[419] Zelezetsky, I., U. Pag, H. G. Sahl, and A. Tossi. 2005. Tuning the biological properties of amphipathic alpha-helical antimicrobial peptides: rational use of minimal amino acid substitutions. *Peptides* 26:2368-76.

[420] Zhang, L., and T. J. Falla. 2006. Antimicrobial Peptides - therapeutic potential *Expert Opin Pharmacother* 7:653-63.

[421] Zhang, L., A. Rozek, and R. E. W. Hancock. 2001. Interaction of cationic antimicrobial peptides with model membranes. *J Biol Chem* 276:35714-22.

[422] Ziere, G. J., M. C. van Dijk, M. K. Bijsterbosch, and T. J. van Berkel. 1992. Lactoferrin uptake by the rat liver. Characterization of the recognition site and effect of selective modification of arginine residues. *J Biol Chem* 267:11229-35.

[423] Zioudrou, C., R. A. Streaty, and W. A. Klee. 1979. Opioid peptides derived from food proteins. The exorphins. *J Biol Chem* 254:2446-9.

[424] Zuccotti, G. V., F. Salvini, E. Riva, and C. Agostoni. 2006. Oral lactoferrin in HIV-1 vertically infected children: an observational follow-up of plasma viral load and immune parameters. *J Int Med Res* 34:88-94.

[425] Zwaal, R. F., and A. J. Schroit. 1997. Pathophysiologic implications of membrane phospholipid asymmetry in blood cells. *Blood* 89:1121-32.

INDEX

A

B

E

F

G

H

I

J

K

L

M

N

O

P

R

S

T

U

V

W

Y

Z